Biologics in Otolaryngology

Editors

NICOLE C. SCHMITT
SARAH K. WISE
ASHKAN MONFARED

OTOLARYNGOLOGIC CLINICS OF NORTH AMERICA

www.oto.theclinics.com

Consulting Editor
SUJANA S. CHANDRASEKHAR

August 2021 • Volume 54 • Number 4

ELSEVIER

1600 John F. Kennedy Boulevard • Suite 1800 • Philadelphia, Pennsylvania, 19103-2899

http://www.oto.theclinics.com

OTOLARYNGOLOGIC CLINICS OF NORTH AMERICA Volume 54, Number 4
August 2021 ISSN 0030-6665, ISBN-13: 978-0-323-83536-7

Editor: Stacy Eastman
Developmental Editor: Diana Ang

Otolaryngologic Clinics of North America (ISSN 0030-6665) is published bimonthly by Elsevier, Inc., 360 Park Avenue South, New York, NY 10010-1710. Months of issue are February, April, June, August, October, and December. Business and Editorial Offices: 1600 John F. Kennedy Blvd., Suite 1800, Philadelphia, PA 19103-2899. Customer Service Office: 6277 Sea Harbor Drive, Orlando, FL 32887-4800. Periodicals postage paid at New York, NY and additional mailing offices. Subscription prices are $437.00 per year (US individuals), $1278.00 per year (US institutions), $100.00 per year (US & Canadian student/resident), $559.00 per year (Canadian individuals), $1348.00 per year (Canadian institutions), $610.00 per year (international individuals), $1348.00 per year (international institutions), $270.00 per year (international student/resident). Foreign air speed delivery is included in all *Clinics*' subscription prices. All prices are subject to change without notice. **POSTMASTER:** Send address changes to *Otolaryngologic Clinics of North America*, Elsevier Health Sciences Division, Subscription Customer Service, 3251 Riverport Lane, Maryland Heights, MO 63043. **Telephone: 1-800-654-2452 (U.S. and Canada); 314-447-8871 (outside U.S. and Canada). Fax: 314-447-8029. E-mail: journalscustomerservice-usa@elsevier.com (for print support); journalsonlinesupport-usa@elsevier.com (for online support).**

Reprints. For copies of 100 or more of articles in this publication, please contact the Commercial Reprints Department, Elsevier Inc., 360 Park Avenue South, New York, NY 10010-1710. Tel.: 212-633-3874; Fax: 212-633-3820; E-mail: reprints@elsevier.com.

Otolaryngologic Clinics of North America is also published in Spanish by McGraw-Hill Interamericana Editores S.A., P.O. Box 5-237, 06500 Mexico D.F., Mexico.

Otolaryngologic Clinics of North America is covered in *MEDLINE/PubMed (Index Medicus), Current Contents/Clinical Medicine, Excerpta Medica, BIOSIS, Science Citation Index,* and *ISI/BIOMED.*

Contributors

CONSULTING EDITOR

SUJANA S. CHANDRASEKHAR, MD, FACS, FAAOHNS
Past President, American Academy of Otolaryngology–Head and Neck Surgery, Secretary-Treasurer, American Otological Society, Partner, ENT & Allergy Associates, LLP, Clinical Professor, Department of Otolaryngology–Head and Neck Surgery, Zucker School of Medicine at Hofstra-Northwell, Hempstead, New York; Clinical Associate Professor, Department of Otolaryngology–Head and Neck Surgery, Icahn School of Medicine at Mount Sinai, New York, New York

EDITORS

NICOLE C. SCHMITT, MD
Associate Professor of Otolaryngology–Head and Neck Surgery, Co-Director for Translational Research, Head and Neck Cancer Program, Winship Cancer Institute, Emory University School of Medicine, Atlanta, Georgia

SARAH K. WISE, MD, MSCR
Professor of Otolaryngology–Head and Neck Surgery, Emory University School of Medicine, Atlanta, Georgia

ASHKAN MONFARED, MD
Associate Professor of Surgery and Neurosurgery, Division of Otolaryngology–Head and Neck Surgery, George Washington University, Washington, DC

JENNIFER A. VILLWOCK, MD, FAAOA
Associate Professor, Department of Otolaryngology–Head Neck Surgery, University of Kansas Medical Center, Kansas City, Kansas

AUTHORS

MONA M. ABAZA, MD, MS
Department of Otolaryngology-Head and Neck Surgery, Vice Chair of Faculty Affairs and Diversity, University of Colorado School of Medicine, Aurora, Colorado

CLINT T. ALLEN, MD, FACS
Chief, Section on Translational Tumor Immunology, National Institute on Deafness and Other Communication Disorders, National Institutes of Health, Bethesda, Maryland

MIRIAM BORNHORST, MD
Department of Pediatric Hematology-Oncology, Gilbert Family Neurofibromatosis Institute, Center for Genetic Medicine Research, Children's National Hospital, Washington, DC

CHRISTOPHER D. BROOK, MD, FAAOA
Associate Professor, Department of Otolaryngology–Head and Neck Surgery, Boston University School of Medicine, Boston, Massachusetts

ZACHARY S. BUCHWALD, MD, PhD
Assistant Professor, Department of Radiation Oncology, Winship Cancer Institute, Emory University School of Medicine, Atlanta, Georgia

CECELIA DAMASK, DO
Lake Mary Ear, Nose, Throat, and Allergy, Lake Mary, Florida

DANIELLA V. DAVIA
Department of Otolaryngology, Zucker School of Medicine at Hofstra-Northwell, Hearing and Speech Center, New Hyde Park, New York

ROBERT L. FERRIS, MD, PhD
Departments of Otolaryngology and Immunology, University of Pittsburgh, UPMC Hillman Cancer Center, Pittsburgh

CHRISTINE FRANZESE, MD
Professor, Director of Allergy, Department of Otolaryngology–Head and Neck Surgery, University of Missouri, Columbia, Missouri

STEVEN A. GORDON, MD, MPH
Otolaryngology–Head and Neck Surgery, University of Utah Health, Salt Lake City, Utah

RICHARD K. GURGEL, MD, MSCI
Otolaryngology–Head and Neck Surgery, University of Utah Health, Salt Lake City, Utah

CHRISTIAN S. HINRICHS, MD
Genitourinary Malignancy Branch, Investigator, Lasker Scholar, National Cancer Institute, Bethesda, Maryland

STELLA E. LEE, MD
Department of Otolaryngology–Head and Neck Surgery, University of Pittsburgh Medical Center, Pittsburgh, Pennsylvania

JOSHUA M. LEVY, MD, MPH
Assistant Professor, Otolaryngology–Head and Neck Surgery, Emory Sinus, Nasal and Allergy Center, Atlanta, Georgia

RAJARSI MANDAL, MD
Department of Otolaryngology–Head and Neck Surgery, Johns Hopkins University, Bloomberg-Kimmel Institute for Cancer Immunotherapy at Johns Hopkins, Baltimore, Maryland

CHRISTOPHER A. MAROUN, MD
Department of Otolaryngology–Head and Neck Surgery, Johns Hopkins University, Bloomberg-Kimmel Institute for Cancer Immunotherapy at Johns Hopkins, Baltimore, Maryland

KATIE MELDER, MD
Department of Otolaryngology–Head and Neck Surgery, University of Pittsburgh Medical Center, Pittsburgh, Pennsylvania

ASHKAN MONFARED, MD
Associate Professor of Surgery and Neurosurgery, Division of Otolaryngology–Head and Neck Surgery, George Washington University, Washington, DC

SCOTT M. NORBERG, DO
Genitourinary Malignancy Branch, Assistant Research Physician, National Cancer Institute, Bethesda, Maryland

VIJAY A. PATEL, MD
Department of Otolaryngology–Head and Neck Surgery, University of Pittsburgh Medical Center, Pittsburgh, Pennsylvania

MICHAEL P. PLATT, MD, MSc, FAAOA
Associate Professor, Department of Otolaryngology–Head and Neck Surgery, Boston University School of Medicine, Boston, Massachusetts

UMA S. RAMASWAMY, MD
Department of Otolaryngology–Head and Neck Surgery, University of Pittsburgh Medical Center, Pittsburgh, Pennsylvania

SCOTT RASKIN, DO
Department of Pediatric Hematology-Oncology, Gilbert Family Neurofibromatosis Institute, Children's National Hospital, Washington, DC

LAUREN T. ROLAND, MD, MSCI
Assistant Professor, Otolaryngology–Head and Neck Surgery, University of California, San Francisco, San Francisco, California

NICOLE C. SCHMITT, MD
Associate Professor of Otolaryngology–Head and Neck Surgery, Co-Director for Translational Research, Head and Neck Cancer Program, Winship Cancer Institute, Emory University School of Medicine, Atlanta, Georgia

SUMITA TRIVEDI, MD
Division of Hematology/Oncology, Department of Medicine, University of Pennsylvania, Philadelphia, Pennsylvania

ANDREA VAMBUTAS, MD, FACS
Department of Otolaryngology, Zucker School of Medicine at Hofstra-Northwell, Hearing and Speech Center, New Hyde Park, New York.

JENNIFER A. VILLWOCK, MD, FAAOA
Associate Professor, Department of Otolaryngology–Head Neck Surgery, Kansas University, University of Kansas Medical Center, Kansas City, Kansas

JULIE L. WEI, MD, FAAP
Division Chief, Pediatric Otolaryngology/Audiology, Director, GME Wellbeing Initiatives, Nemours Children's Hospital, Chair, Otolaryngology Education, Professor, Otolaryngology–Head and Neck Surgery, University of Central Florida College of Medicine, Orlando, Florida

SARAH K. WISE, MD, MSCR
Professor of Otolaryngology–Head and Neck Surgery, Emory University School of Medicine, Atlanta, Georgia

Contents

Foreword: Benefiting Otolaryngology Patients with Biologics **xiii**

Sujana S. Chandrasekhar

Preface: Biologics in Otolaryngology: Triumphs, Challenges, and New Possibilities **xv**

Nicole C. Schmitt, Sarah K. Wise, and Ashkan Monfared

Biologics in Otolaryngology: Past, Present, and Future **675**

Nicole C. Schmitt, Ashkan Monfared, and Sarah K. Wise

Biologics have been widely adopted in multiple subspecialties of otolaryngology. This article provides an overview of past, present, and future uses of biologics in otolaryngology with emphasis on allergic rhinitis, chronic rhinosinusitis with polyposis, head and neck squamous cell carcinoma, salivary and skull base tumors, hearing loss, and other otologic disorders.

Current Evidence for Biologic Therapy in Chronic Rhinosinusitis with Nasal Polyposis **689**

Uma S. Ramaswamy, Katie Melder, Vijay A. Patel, and Stella E. Lee

The problem surrounding the management of chronic rhinosinusitis with nasal polyposis (CRSwNP) has captivated practitioners for over 2 millennia. Although this the current paradigms such as topical medications including intranasal corticosteroids and saline irrigations; systemic drugs such as oral corticosteroids and antimicrobials for symptomatic flares; and functional endoscopic sinus surgery is are effective for most individuals with CRSwNP, there remains a subset of patients with recalcitrant disease that is difficult to control. With the advent of biologic agents, targeted disease and cell-specific therapy have become available for various immune-mediated conditions.

Choosing the Right Patient for Biologic Therapy in Chronic Rhinosinusitis with Nasal Polyposis: Endotypes, Patient Characteristics, and Defining Failures of Standard Therapy **701**

Michael P. Platt and Christopher D. Brook

There are many phenotypes of chronic sinusitis and clinical variables that differ between patients. The ability to accurately diagnose, predict prognosis, and select the appropriate treatment depends on the understanding of disease endotypes. Chronic sinusitis is in the early stages of disease endotyping. The ability to identify endotypes is at the forefront of clinical research. Endotyping of chronic sinusitis uses clinical information, radiographic studies, and pathophysiologic data. Understanding of the full spectrum of chronic sinusitis is in its infancy. A personalized approach to treatment will consider standard medical therapies, sinus surgeries, and targeted use of biologic agents.

Knowledge Gaps and Research Needs for Biologic Therapy in Rhinology Practice 709

Lauren T. Roland and Joshua M. Levy

Biologic agents are emerging for chronic rhinosinusitis with nasal polyposis (CRSwNP) patients with recalcitrant disease. Although early work has shown promise, and several trials are ongoing, there is significant work to be done in this field. CRS patients form a heterogeneous group, and identification of appropriate patients for the use of biologic agents is critical. The determination of endotype-specific biomarkers will help define patient selection and predict treatment response. As more biologic agents become approved, head-to-head trials will be needed to compare them with similar products. Ultimately, cost-effectiveness analyses and further quality of life studies will guide treatment recommendations.

Mechanisms and Practical Use of Biologic Therapies for Allergy and Asthma Indications 717

Cecelia Damask and Christine Franzese

This article presents a concise overview of the important aspects of the immunologic mechanisms targeted by T-helper 2–directed monoclonal antibodies, as well as their practical applications in the treatment of allergic disorders (specifically allergic rhinitis) and asthma. Several of these novel agents treat multiple diseases, so understanding their targets and the underlying disease process can aid patient selection. In addition, the particular targets of the therapeutics seem to be shifting to include not only agents that intervene against inflammatory cytokines or their receptors but also specific molecular epitopes and cellular surface proteins.

Immunotherapeutic Strategies for Head and Neck Cancer 729

Zachary S. Buchwald and Nicole C. Schmitt

Immunotherapy has revolutionized the treatment of cancer, including head and neck squamous cell carcinoma (HNSCC). Most immune therapies consist of biologics, including monoclonal antibodies, vaccines, and cell therapy. This article reviews basic tumor immunology and provides an overview of immunotherapeutic strategies used for HNSCC. The current indications for use of programmed cell death protein 1 immune checkpoint inhibitors in recurrent/metastatic HNSCC are summarized. In addition, new immunotherapeutic biologics and combinations under investigation in early-phase clinical trials are highlighted.

Epidermal Growth Factor Receptor-Targeted Therapy for Head and Neck Cancer 743

Sumita Trivedi and Robert L. Ferris

The epidermal growth factor receptor (EGFR) is an important therapeutic target in head and neck squamous cell carcinomas (HNSCCs). EGFR-targeted agents including monoclonal antibodies and tyrosine kinase inhibitors have shown mixed results in clinical trials. To date, only cetuximab, an anti-EGFR monoclonal antibody, is approved for use in local/regional advanced and recurrent or metastatic HNSCC. This article reviews the mechanism of action of cetuximab and its antitumor immune effects and the data to support its use in HNSCC. It additionally provides an

overview of other EGFR monoclonal antibodies and small molecule tyrosine kinase inhibitors that have been studied.

Anti-PD-1 Immune Checkpoint Blockade for Head and Neck Cancer: Biomarkers of Response and Resistance 751

Christopher A. Maroun and Rajarsi Mandal

Immunotherapy in recent years has solidified its position as the fourth pillar of cancer treatment alongside surgery, chemotherapy, and radiation. Although in its infancy, when compared with these other conventional therapeutic strategies, immunotherapy has provided a chance for prolonged survival, and in some cases even cure, for patients who previously would have been given a terminal diagnosis. In this article, the various mechanisms of resistance to immunotherapy and biomarkers of response that have so far been explored in the literature are outlined.

Advances in Adoptive Cell Therapy for Head and Neck Cancer 761

Scott M. Norberg and Christian S. Hinrichs

This article reviews the most recent literature describing clinical advances in adoptive cell therapy for patients with head and neck cancer. Clinical trials with tumor-infiltrating lymphocyte and gene-engineered T-cell receptor T-cell therapy are highlighted.

Biologics for the Treatment of Recurrent Respiratory Papillomatosis 769

Clint T. Allen

This article aims to educate readers on adjuvant therapies for recurrent respiratory papillomatosis (RRP). Although antivirals are injected locally into papillomas as an adjuvant treatment, new biologics targeting vascular endothelial growth factor or induction of human papillomavirus (HPV)-specific immunity are gaining traction with demonstration of clinical benefit and mechanism of action in retrospective case series and prospective clinical trials. The future of RRP treatment, alone or in combination with surgery, lies in the careful clinical study of vascular and immune targeting agents that balance the risk of adverse events with the chance for elimination of HPV-infected cells.

Past and Future Biologics for Otologic Disorders 779

Steven A. Gordon and Richard K. Gurgel

Biologic therapies have the ability to fundamentally change the management of hearing loss; clinicians need to familiarize themselves with their prospective applications in practice. This article reviews the current application of 4 categories of biological therapeutics—growth factors, apoptosis inhibitors, monoclonal antibodies, and gene therapy—in otology and their potential future directions and applications.

Biological Treatments of Neurofibromatosis Type 2 and Other Skull Base Disorders 789

Scott Raskin and Miriam Bornhorst

Studies of genomic alterations that occur in skull base tumors have provided information regarding biological aberrations that are necessary for the growth and maintenance of these tumors. This has led to the

development and initiation of clinical trials incorporating biological treatments for many skull base tumors. The exciting developments of molecularly targeted therapy for the treatment of skull base tumors may provide noninvasive therapeutic options for patients that can be used either alone or in combination with surgery and/or radiation therapy. Future analysis and continued scientific discovery of treatments for skull base tumors can lead to improved outcomes in patients.

Biologics for Immune-Mediated Sensorineural Hearing Loss **803**

Andrea Vambutas and Daniella V. Davia

Immune-mediated hearing losses include autoimmune inner ear disease, sudden sensorineural hearing loss, and Meniere's disease. Standard therapy for an acute decline in hearing is timely use of corticosteroids. Although 60% to 70% of patients are initially corticosteroid-responsive, that responsiveness is lost over time. In corticosteroid-resistant patients, increased expression of interleukin (IL)-1 is observed, and these patients may benefit from IL-1 inhibition. Autoinflammatory diseases are characterized by dysregulation of the innate immune response, clinically include sensorineural hearing loss, and benefit from IL-1 inhibition, thereby further establishing the relationship of IL-1 with immune-mediated sensorineural hearing loss.

Special Article Series: Intentionally Shaping the Future of Otolaryngology

Foreword: Building the Future We Wish to See **xvii**

Sujana S. Chandrasekhar

Preface: From Crisis to Change **xxi**

Jennifer A. Villwock

Women in Academic Medicine and Leadership **815**

Mona M. Abaza

Women lag in leadership roles in many fields, but in academic medicine, and particularly in Otolaryngology, women are even further behind. Understanding personal and cultural biases, changing institutional and systemic practices that perpetuate the challenges, and developing and supporting individual skills will all be necessary to improve the representation of women leaders in academic medicine.

Balance Versus Integration: Work-Life Considerations **823**

Julie L. Wei and Jennifer A. Villwock

The term work-life balance may cause physicians to feel inadequate in pursuing a reality in which work and life each have equal importance. Furthermore, the term implies competition between these 2 realms. Instead, work-life integration is a more constructive and realistic term. Achieving harmonious integration requires self-reflection on the current state, goals, and resources and strategies needed to achieve and maintain such a state. Prioritizing aspects of both, and aligning them with individual requirements, while incorporating consistent and intentional investment of time and efforts in both professional and personal arenas is crucial to cultivate and sustain longitudinal well-being.

OTOLARYNGOLOGIC CLINICS OF NORTH AMERICA

FORTHCOMING ISSUES

October 2021
The Dizzy Patient
Maja Svrakic and Meredith E. Adams, *Editors*

December 2021
Childhood Hearing Loss
Nancy M. Young and Anne Marie Tharpe, *Editors*

February 2022
Business of Otolaryngology: 2022
Stephen Paul Cragle and Eileen H. Dauer, *Editors*

RECENT ISSUES

June 2021
Modern Approach to the Salivary Glands
William R. Ryan and M. Boyd Gillespie, *Editors*

April 2021
Head and Neck Cutaneous Cancer
Cecelia E. Schmalbach and Kelly M. Malloy, *Editors*

February 2021
Endoscopic Ear Surgery
Manuela X. Fina, Justin S. Golub, Daniel J. Lee, *Editors*

Foreword
Benefiting Otolaryngology Patients with Biologics

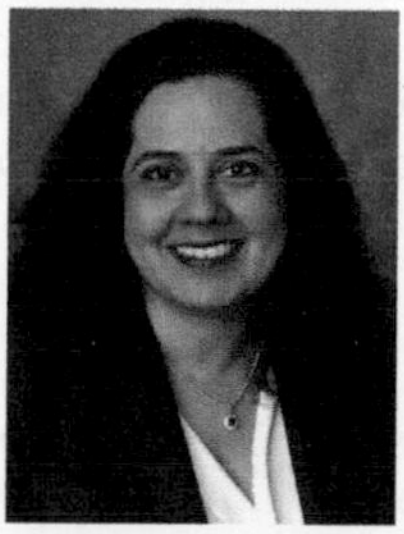

Sujana S. Chandrasekhar, MD, FACS, FAAOHNS
Consulting Editor

Biologics, or biological medications, are used to prevent, treat, and cure disease. These drugs are developed from blood, proteins, viruses, and living organisms and from a variety of living sources, including mammals, birds, insects, plants, and bacteria. They can be made of tiny components like sugars, proteins, or DNA, or can be from whole cells or tissues. They have been used commonly in Medicine. We are all familiar with the biological medications such as Botox (botulinum toxin or onabotulinumtoxina) used for muscle tension, migraines, and wrinkles, and Lantus (long-acting insulin or insulin glargine) used for diabetes mellitus. Many of us are aware of other biologics, such as Humira (adalimumab), Remicade (infliximab), Rituxan (rituximab), and Enbrel (etanercept), which are used to treat rheumatoid arthritis and other autoimmune diseases, such as psoriasis and Crohn disease.

Introduced relatively recently in Otolaryngology, the biologics with which we are most comfortable are used for refractory chronic rhinosinusitis with nasal polyposis (CRSwNP). Biologic therapy with targeted activity within the type 2 inflammatory pathway can improve clinical signs and symptoms in patients with CRSwNP that persist despite medical therapy and endoscopic sinus surgery. Expanding from there, we have data regarding the utility of biological medications in other aspects of our field, including rhinitis, asthma and allergy, laryngology, head and neck oncology, otology, and neurotology, as you will learn in this comprehensive issue of *Otolaryngologic Clinics of North America* on Biologics in Otolaryngology. Biologics can reduce the need for aggressive surgery in conditions such as recurrent respiratory papillomatosis and extensive squamous cell carcinoma and may prevent progression of hearing loss in autoimmune ear disease and limit tumor growth and sequelae in neurofibromatosis.

Because they are derived from such diverse sources, the manufacture of biologics is more complicated than for other drugs. They are harder to purify, process, and produce, and once formulated, biologics tend to be more unpredictable and can be

Otolaryngol Clin N Am 54 (2021) xiii–xiv
https://doi.org/10.1016/j.otc.2021.05.022
0030-6665/21/© 2021 Published by Elsevier Inc.

more susceptible to light and temperature. The work to show efficacy for various conditions is likewise more involved; the reader is benefiting from decades of translational research.

I commend Guest Editors Drs Sarah K. Wise, Ashkan Monfared, and Nicole Schmitt, for tackling this challenging subject and compiling an outstanding group of articles and authors. The reader is treated to this single resource that contains up-to-date information on the current utility of biologics in Otolaryngology, as well as the future potential of this class of agents. Addition of biologics to our armamentarium allows otolaryngologic care to advance along the spectrum of interventions from open to minimally invasive surgery, and from surgery alone to collaboration with medical experts in medical and radiation oncology and pharmacology, in order to optimize patient outcomes.

Sujana S. Chandrasekhar, MD, FACS, FAAOHNS
Consulting Editor
Otolaryngologic Clinics of North America
Past President, American Academy of
Otolaryngology–Head and Neck Surgery
Secretary-Treasurer, American Otological Society
Partner, ENT & Allergy Associates, LLP
18 East 48th Street, 2nd Floor
New York, NY 10017, USA

Clinical Professor, Department of Otolaryngology–
Head and Neck Surgery
Zucker School of Medicine at
Hofstra-Northwell
Hempstead, NY, USA

Clinical Associate Professor
Department of Otolaryngology–
Head and Neck Surgery
Icahn School of Medicine at Mount Sinai
New York, NY, USA

E-mail address:
ssc@nyotology.com

Website:
http://www.ears.nyc

Preface
Biologics in Otolaryngology: Triumphs, Challenges, and New Possibilities

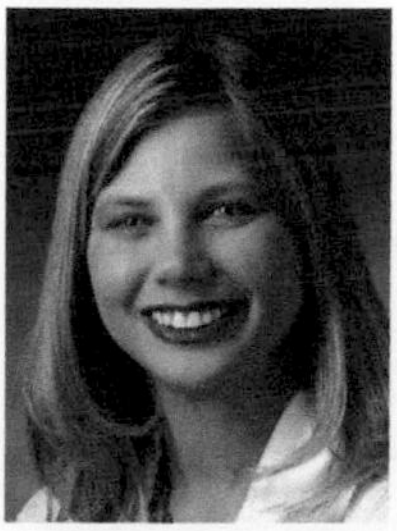
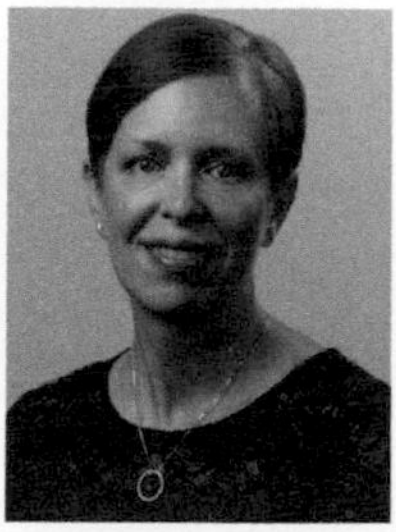
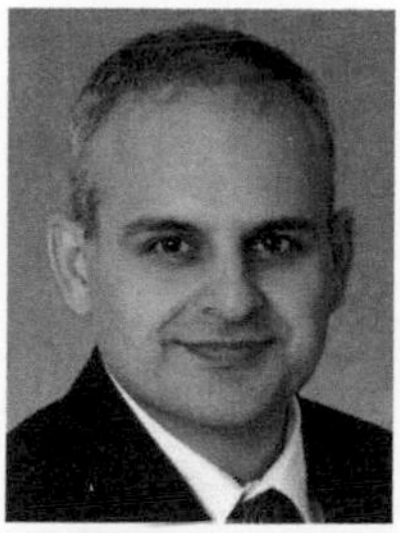

Nicole C. Schmitt, MD   Sarah K. Wise, MD   Ashkan Monfared, MD
Editors

Therapeutic agents derived from living sources, including microorganisms, plants, animals, and humans, are known as "biologics." These agents have had a major impact on all subspecialties of otolaryngology in recent decades. For example, botulinum toxin has diverse applications in laryngology, facial plastic surgery, and the treatment of some salivary gland disorders. Monoclonal antibodies targeting specific cytokines have become indispensable to rhinologists for the treatment of nasal polyposis. Exciting advancements in head and neck oncology have centered on monoclonal antibodies targeting immune checkpoints, such as programmed cell death-1. A variety of growth factors, anti-inflammatory biologics, and gene therapies have been explored for hearing loss and other otologic disorders.

In this issue of *Otolaryngologic Clinics of North America*, we begin with an overview article highlighting some of the major advances in the use of biologics in otolaryngology. The next section highlights current evidence on the use of biologics for nasal polyposis and other allergic diseases. The next several articles summarize current practices and future directions in the use of biologics for neoplastic diseases of the head and neck, including recurrent respiratory papillomatosis and head and neck squamous cell carcinoma. Since immunotherapy is the most rapidly evolving area in head and neck oncology, one article provides an overview on immunotherapeutic strategies, followed by articles with more detailed information on cetuximab, resistance to immune checkpoint blockade, and adoptive cell therapy. The final section begins with an overview of biologics used for otologic diseases, followed by two more articles on biologics for skull-base diseases (with a focus on neurofibromatosis type II) and autoimmune ear disease. One of our aims in this issue was to provide practical information that applies to current patient care, but we also highlight exciting areas of ongoing

Otolaryngol Clin N Am 54 (2021) xv–xvi
https://doi.org/10.1016/j.otc.2021.05.021
0030-6665/21/© 2021 Published by Elsevier Inc.

investigation in the use of biologics. Decades of translational research in otolaryngology have led to the advent of these agents, enabling us to take better care of our patients.

Nicole C. Schmitt, MD
Emory Department of Otolaryngology–
Head and Neck Surgery
550 Peachtree Street
MOT Suite 1135
Atlanta, GA 30308, USA

Sarah K. Wise, MD
Emory Department of Otolaryngology–
Head and Neck Surgery
550 Peachtree Street
MOT Suite 1135
Atlanta, GA 30308, USA

Ashkan Monfared, MD
Medical Faculty Associates at
George Washington University
Division of Otolaryngology–
Head and Neck Surgery
2300 M Street, NW, 4th Floor
Washington, DC 20037, USA

E-mail addresses:
nicole.cherie.schmitt@emory.edu (N.C. Schmitt)
skmille@emory.edu (S.K. Wise)
amonfared@mfa.gwu.edu (A. Monfared)

Biologics in Otolaryngology

Past, Present, and Future

Nicole C. Schmitt, MD[a,*], Ashkan Monfared, MD[b],
Sarah K. Wise, MD, MSCR[c]

KEYWORDS

• Biologics • Monoclonal antibodies • Immunotherapy • Otolaryngology • Cancer
• Allergy • Rhinosinusitis • Nasal polyposis

KEY POINTS

- Biologics are medicines derived from living sources, including vaccines, monoclonal antibodies, serum or blood cells, gene therapies, and toxins.
- Targeted therapies have shown substantial benefit for chronic rhinosinusitis with nasal polyposis and other T-helper-2–mediated respiratory diseases relevant to otolaryngology.
- Immune checkpoint blockade has revolutionized the treatment of recurrent/metastatic head and neck cancers.
- Immune modulators are providing exciting treatments for conditions such as neurofibromatosis type II and autoimmune-mediated ear disorders for which there have been few optimal treatment options previously.

INTRODUCTION

Advancements in the use of biologics have dramatically improved the ability to treat many clinical conditions in otolaryngology. Therapeutic agents classified as biologics include any biomedical agents derived from living sources, including microorganisms, plants, and animals (including humans).[1] The use of biologics for the treatment of disease may date as far back as 1000 BC, in the form of variolation for smallpox.[2] In the present era, biologics in clinical use include vaccines, blood products (including cells), monoclonal antibodies targeting specific molecular pathways, nanotherapies, gene therapies, toxins, and antitoxins.[2] Biologic agents are used daily in otolaryngology, spanning all subspecialties: botulinum toxin in laryngology and facial plastic surgery;

[a] Head and Neck Cancer Program, Department of Otolaryngology – Head and Neck Surgery, Winship Cancer Institute, Emory University School of Medicine, 550 Peachtree Street Northeast, 11th Floor Otolaryngology, Atlanta, GA 30308, USA; [b] Division of Otolaryngology – Head and Neck Surgery, George Washington University, Washington, DC 20052, USA; [c] Department of Otolaryngology – Head and Neck Surgery, Emory University School of Medicine, 550 Peachtree Street Northeast, 11th Floor Otolaryngology, Atlanta, GA 30308, USA
* Corresponding author.
E-mail address: nicole.cherie.schmitt@emory.edu

Otolaryngol Clin N Am 54 (2021) 675–687
https://doi.org/10.1016/j.otc.2021.04.001
oto.theclinics.com

biologics targeting immunoglobulin (Ig) E or cytokines in rhinology; immune checkpoint blockade for head and neck cancer; and biologics for hearing loss and other otologic disorders. This article provides an overview of current and future uses for biologics in otolaryngology head and neck surgery. Updates and further details on the use of biologics for specific subspecialty areas are highlighted elsewhere in this issue.

DISCUSSION

Immune Modulators for Rhinology and Otology

Biologics for T-helper 2–mediated respiratory indications, with a focus on nasal polyposis and allergic rhinitis

There are 5 biologic therapies currently approved for respiratory diseases that are on the T-helper (Th) 2 inflammatory spectrum (**Table 1**). Therefore, several important mediators of the Th2 inflammatory cascade provide targets for these biologics (**Fig. 1**). A brief overview of the important aspects of Th2-mediated respiratory inflammation is included here, with the aim to provide a basic immunologic understanding for clinical practitioners who may prescribe these biologic therapies. In-depth discussion of the current status of the evidence for biologics for nasal polyposis, patient selection for biologic therapy in nasal polyposis, and biologic therapy for allergy and asthma indications are also included in this issue.

Immunology summary. When a naive T cell is exposed to interleukin (IL)-4 during T-cell priming, it can undergo differentiation into a Th2 cell.[3] Th2 cells influence B-cell class switching to IgE, producing cells by secreting IL-4, IL-5, and IL-13.[4] When mast cell–bound IgE is cross-linked by a recognized allergen, mast cell degranulation ensues and various mediators are released, including histamine, tryptase, cytokines, leukotrienes, prostaglandins, and proteases. Acting on the respiratory mucosa and smooth muscle lining, symptomatic effects of these mast cell mediators may include increased mucus secretion, bronchoconstriction, and vascular permeability with subsequent edema, itching, and other symptoms typical of allergic rhinitis and allergic asthma. Th2 cells also produce IL-5. IL-5 influences maturation of eosinophils in the bone marrow, as well as their release into the bloodstream. IL-5 also affects eosinophil and basophil growth, maturation activation, and survival. Furthermore, eosinophils produce IL-5, creating an autocrine feedback loop.[5] Mediators released by eosinophils contribute to bronchial hyperreactivity and bronchoconstriction, mucus hypersecretion, tissue damage and airway remodeling, and increased asthma exacerbations.[6,7] Eosinophils are also frequently identified in chronic rhinosinusitis with nasal polyposis (CRSwNP), with increased eosinophil counts linked to polyp recurrence after sinus surgery, higher rates of revision surgery, and suggestion of a more aggressive surgical approach.[8–11] Targets of currently available Th2 respiratory biologic therapies include IgE, IL-5 and its α receptor, as well as the IL-4 α receptor, which is shared by IL-4 and IL-13.

Omalizumab (anti–immunoglobulin E). Omalizumab is an anti-IgE biologic therapy that was initially approved by the US Food and Drug Administration (FDA) to treat asthma in 2003, making it the first respiratory biologic therapy on the market. It is indicated for moderate to severe persistent asthma in patients 6 years of age and older. The asthma must be inadequately controlled with inhaled corticosteroid therapy, and patients must have reactivity to a perennial aeroallergen by skin or in vitro allergy testing. For asthma, omalizumab is administered subcutaneously, with dosing based on serum total IgE level and the patient's weight. Omalizumab is also indicated for chronic idiopathic urticaria in patients 12 years of age and older who have persistent

Table 1
Biologic therapies available for T-helper 2–mediated respiratory indications, 2020

Biologic Name Trade Name	Target	Source of Biologic	Effects	Indications, Age (y)	Method of Administration
Dupilumab Dupixent	IL-4Rα	Humanized monoclonal IgG4 antibody	Binds to IL4Rα subunit (shared by IL-4 and IL-13) Inhibits IL-4 signaling (type I receptor) and IL-4 + IL-13 (type II receptor)	Atopic dermatitis (moderate-severe), ≥6 Asthma (moderate to severe), ≥12 Nasal polyposis, ≥18	Subcutaneous
Omalizumab Xolair	IgE	Recombinant DNA-derived humanized IgG1κ monoclonal Ab	Binds to free IgE Inhibits IgE binding to FcεR1 receptors on mast cells/basophils Reduces FcεR1 IgE receptors on basophils	Asthma (moderate to severe persistent, with perennial IgE-mediated allergy), ≥6 Chronic idiopathic urticaria, ≥12 Nasal polyposis, ≥18	Subcutaneous
Mepolizumab Nucala	IL-5	Recombinant DNA-derived humanized IgG1κ monoclonal Ab	Binds to IL-5 Blocks binding of IL-5 to IL-5Rα Dose-dependent decrease in blood eosinophils	Asthma (severe, eosinophilic), ≥6 Eosinophilic granulomatosis with polyangiitis (EGPA, formerly Churg-Strauss syndrome), ≥12	Subcutaneous
Reslizumab Cinquair	IL-5	Recombinant DNA-derived humanized IgG4κ monoclonal Ab	Binds to IL-5 Blocks binding of IL-5 to IL-5Rα Dose-dependent decrease in blood eosinophils	Asthma (severe, eosinophilic), ≥18	Intravenous
Benralizumab Fasenra	IL-5Rα	Humanized monoclonal IgG1κ Ab	Binds to IL-5Rα on eosinophils Draws NK cells to encourage cell death Blood eosinophils reduced Blood basophils reduced	Asthma (severe, eosinophilic), ≥12	Subcutaneous

Abbreviations: Ab, antibody; IL, interleukin; NK, natural killer.

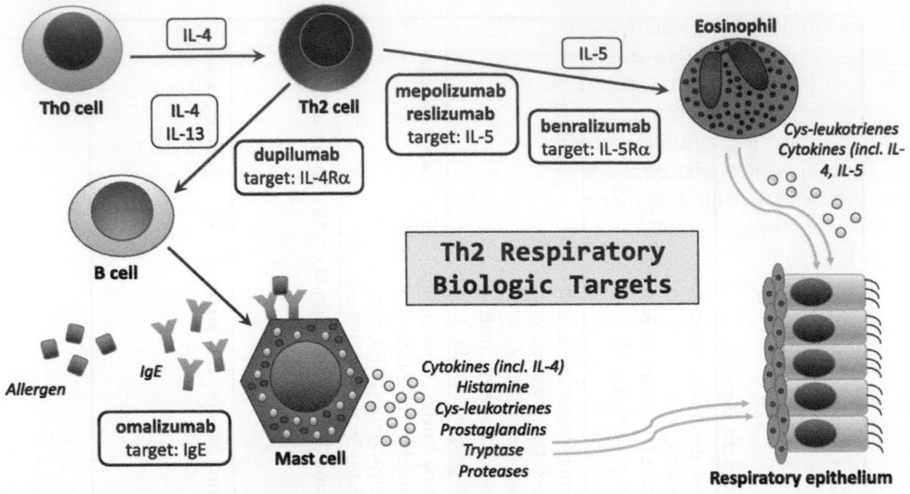

Fig. 1. Respiratory biologic targets. IL, interleukin.

symptoms despite appropriate antihistamine treatment. For chronic idiopathic urticaria, omalizumab is also dosed subcutaneously but does not require IgE or weight-based calculations. In December 2020, omalizumab was approved by the FDA as add-on maintenance therapy for nasal polyposis for patients 18 years and older who have inadequate response to nasal corticosteroids. Similar to asthma, omalizumab dosing for nasal polyposis is based on serum total IgE and patient weight. It is given every 2 to 4 weeks.

Some otolaryngologists who treat asthma and urticaria may prescribe omalizumab; however, allergic rhinitis is more commonly treated in the otolaryngology practice. Omalizumab has been assessed via randomized controlled trials for efficacy in allergic rhinitis caused by ragweed pollen,[12] birch pollen,[13] Japanese cedar pollen,[14] as well as perennial allergens.[15] A systematic review assessing symptom scores, rescue medication use, and quality of life in allergic rhinitis revealed that omalizumab was superior to placebo and was generally well tolerated.[16] Furthermore, studies of combination therapy with omalizumab and inhalant allergen immunotherapy have shown decreased symptoms and decreased mediation use compared with omalizumab or immunotherapy alone.[17–19] These results are supportive of the benefit of omalizumab in allergic rhinitis, which follows its IgE-blocking mechanism of action. However, omalizumab does not have a clinical indication for allergic rhinitis and is not routinely used for this purpose.

In the realm of nasal polyposis, recent randomized controlled trials (POLYP1 [n = 138] and POLYP2 [n = 127] studies) have shown benefit with omalizumab in adults with CRSwNP who are refractory to intranasal corticosteroids. Following a 24-week application of omalizumab versus placebo, omalizumab showed benefit in nasal polyp score, nasal congestion score, rhinorrhea and postnasal drip scores, olfaction measures (loss of smell score, University of Pennsylvania Smell Identification Test), quality of life (Sinonasal Outcome Test [SNOT-22]), Total Nasal Symptoms Score (TNSS), and need for surgery.[20] At the time of this writing, omalizumab has recently received FDA approval for nasal polyposis.

Mepolizumab and reslizumab (anti–interleukin -5) and benralizumab (anti–interleukin-5Rα). The group of biologic therapies that affects IL-5 includes mepolizumab (anti–IL-5), reslizumab (anti–IL-5), and benralizumab (anti–IL-5Rα). All 3 are indicated for severe eosinophilic asthma. Mepolizumab and benralizumab may be used to treat asthma in patients 12 years of age and older, whereas reslizumab may be used in patients aged 18 years and older. Mepolizumab is also indicated to treat eosinophilic granulomatosis with polyangiitis (EGPA; formerly Churg-Strauss syndrome), which can be a cause of recalcitrant CRSwNP along with additional systemic vasculitic manifestations. In clinical practice, mepolizumab and benralizumab are administered via subcutaneous injection; reslizumab is administered via intravenous infusion.

Biologics that target IL-5 have been studied in CRSwNP, although none are FDA-approved for this indication as of November 2020. The earliest study of mepolizumab, given intravenously in 30 patients refractory to corticosteroid therapy, revealed that patients receiving mepolizumab had a significant reduction in nasal polyp size compared with placebo.[21] A subsequent intravenous mepolizumab study of 105 patients showed improvement in nasal polyp score, symptoms, patient-reported outcome measures (SNOT-22), olfaction, and need for surgery.[22] The SYNAPSE study of subcutaneously administered mepolizumab for CRSwNP is a completed phase 3 trial that enrolled patients with a history of prior sinus surgery who were in need of further surgery because of polyp recurrence. Although results of this study have not been published in the scientific literature or posted on clinicaltrials.gov as of November 2020, media outlets report that the study met both of its coprimary end points, with significant improvement in nasal polyp score and nasal obstruction.[23] Reslizumab has been investigated via subgroup analysis that included patients with CRSwNP receiving this biologic therapy in a larger study of patients with asthma. The results of this investigation showed that patients with CRSwNP receiving reslizumab had an 83% reduction in clinical asthma exacerbations, which was significantly lower than placebo.[24]

Benralizumab has also been studied in CRSwNP. A recent small observational study showed beneficial effects of benralizumab in SNOT-22 score, endoscopic polyp score, Lund-Mackay score, and blood eosinophil count.[25] In addition, post hoc pooled analysis of the phase 3 SIROCCO and CALIMA asthma trials revealed that patients with nasal polyposis had higher mean blood eosinophil counts and greater baseline mean oral corticosteroid use than patients without nasal polyposis. Study outcomes for the benralizumab treatment group in patients with nasal polyps were enhanced for patients with nasal polyps, including reduced exacerbation rates, increased forced expiratory volume in 1 second, improved asthma symptom scores, and improved asthma quality of life scores.[26] As noted on clinicaltrials.gov, phase 3 studies of benralizumab in CRSwNP are either completed or recruiting, although no results have been published in the scientific literature or posted on clinical trials sites as of November 2020. Media outlets report that the OSTRO phase 3 trial has met its coprimary end points of nasal polyp score and nasal obstruction.[27]

Dupilumab (anti–interleukin -4Rα). Dupilumab is a humanized monoclonal antibody that blocks the IL-4 α-receptor subunit. This receptor subunit can be bound by IL-4 and IL-13, which results in substantial immunologic effects in the Th2 inflammatory cascade. Dupilumab is indicated as add-on therapy for moderate to severe asthma that is eosinophilic in cause or oral corticosteroid–dependent in patients aged 12 years or older. Dupilumab is also indicated for patients 6 years of age or older who have moderate to severe atopic dermatitis refractory or intolerant to prescription topical therapies. In addition, dupilumab is approved as add-on therapy to treat CRSwNP not controlled with standard medications. For nasal polyposis, dupilumab is approved for patients 18 years of age and older. Although specific dosing varies by indication, dupilumab is administered subcutaneously.

The pivotal studies supporting the FDA approval of dupilumab for CRSwNP were double-blind, placebo-controlled, randomized controlled trials known as LIBERTY NP SINUS-24 (n = 276) and LIBERTY SINUS-52 (n = 448).[28] These trials enrolled adults with bilateral nasal polyposis refractory to intranasal corticosteroids, who had received systemic corticosteroids in the 2 years before the study, or had sinonasal surgery. The dupilumab groups had significant improvement in coprimary end points including nasal polyp score and nasal congestion/obstruction score. There were also significant benefits of dupilumab on several secondary end points, including Lund-Mackay computed tomography score, total symptom score, measures of olfaction, and quality of life (SNOT-22). Of note, when patients were discontinued from dupilumab and observed, measures such as nasal polyp score and nasal congestion/obstruction score returned to levels close to baseline. On subgroup analysis of nonsteroidal antiinflammatory drug–exacerbated respiratory disease (28% of the cohort), in patients with prior sinonasal surgery (58%–74% of the cohort) and patients with comorbid asthma (59% of the cohort), improvements with dupilumab were similar to the overall treatment population. The most common adverse events included nasopharyngitis, headache, epistaxis, worsening of polyps/asthma, and injection site reactions and were more common in the placebo group. It should also be noted that some patients on dupilumab show increased blood eosinophil levels, with the potential for unmasking EGPA; therefore, symptoms of joint pain, neuropathy, and other aspects of EGPA should be monitored. In June 2019, dupilumab was granted FDA approval for treatment of CRSwNP.

Biologics for otologic diseases

The advent of biologics for treatment of rhinologic disorders will have an indirect, but significant, effect on otologic disorders as well. Because much of chronic middle ear disorder is caused by mucosal disease lining the upper aerodigestive tract, biologic treatments designed for allergic rhinitis and nasal polyposis would ameliorate a large segment of otologic disorders. However, there are a few areas where biologics are set to revolutionize century-old treatments in otology.

Tympanic membrane regeneration. One such exciting new treatment strategy is nonsurgical correction of tympanic membrane perforations. Little has changed in terms of surgical management of tympanic membrane perforations over the past 70 years.[29] Whether using homograft or allograft materials, or performing a medial or lateral graft technique, 1 thing has remained the same: surgery remains the only method for correction of chronic tympanic membrane perforations. Use of human-derived growth factors is one of the greatest leaps in otology, possibly since the inception of cochlear implantation.[30] Two major contenders, epidermal growth factor (EGF) and basic fibroblast growth factor (bFGF or FGF-2), have been used in numerous human trials. In a recent meta-analysis of 14 studies, which included a total of 1072 patients, bFGF was found to significantly improve the closure rate of tympanic membrane perforations, although it did not show any difference in hearing outcomes.[31] Similarly, since its earliest utility in the animal model,[32] EGF has been the subject of human trials as well.[33] Most recently heparin-binding epidermal growth factor–like growth factor was shown to facilitate healing of subacute tympanic membrane perforations better than both EGF and b-FGF.[34]

Sensorineural hearing loss. Affecting some half a billion of the world's population, hearing loss affects about 10% to 14% of humanity sometime in their lifetimes. Almost all of these are adults with sensorineural hearing loss.[35,36] It is no surprise that dozens of new biotechnology and pharmaceutical companies are racing to develop new therapeutics for sensorineural hearing loss.[37] From a clinical standpoint, these efforts are targeting otoprotection, regeneration of hair cells, reduction of tinnitus, improvement of balance disorders, and central hearing disorders. They use a wide variety of methods, including novel and repurposed drugs, gene therapy using RNA interference or variety of vectors, and stem cell treatment. These efforts are discussed in greater detail elsewhere in this issue.

Autoimmune ear disease. Perhaps in no other part of otology would the effect of new biologics be as dramatic as in treatment of autoimmune ear disorders. Group together based on their transient response to corticosteroid, these conditions lack a uniform and precise definition. With no identified biologic marker or diagnostic tests, these disorders have similarly eluded efficacious treatment options. Even corticosteroids, by response to which these conditions are defined, eventually cease to provide any improvement in a large proportion of these patients. That is why the new generations of biologics are poised to advance not only the treatment but also the understanding of these disorders. Both adaptive and innate immune mechanisms have been implicated in these disorders.[38] Autoantibodies, as well as upregulation of cytokines such as IL-1 and tumor necrosis factor (TNF), have been described in animal and human studies.[39–41] Strum and colleagues[42] recently performed a systematic review of pharmacotherapy for these disorders, including the biologics used systematically or through intratympanic administration. Although some, such as ankarina (IL-1 antagonist) and 2 TNF antagonists (golimumab and infliximab) showed some promise, all studies were done in a limited number of patients.[42] These modalities are discussed in greater detail elsewhere in this issue. It is likely that, based on the select response to the therapeutic effects of these new biologics, distinct disorders will be identified and their pathophysiology better elucidated.

Biologics for Neoplastic Diseases in Otolaryngology

Over the past 2 decades, the use of biologics has dramatically improved the treatment and understanding of neoplastic disease in otolaryngology, including head and neck squamous cell carcinoma (HNSCC), recurrent respiratory papillomatosis, and tumors of the skull base and/or salivary glands. The approval of immune checkpoint inhibitors, in particular, has revolutionized the treatment of HNSCC and other cancers.

Biologics for head and neck squamous cell carcinoma

The first biologic agent approved for HNSCC was cetuximab, a monoclonal antibody targeting epidermal growth factor receptor (EGFR). Cetuximab is a chimeric mouse-human IgG antibody, and responses correlate with an acneiform skin rash that is thought to be immune mediated. Interestingly, clinical trials of other EGFR inhibitors have been disappointing. Further, cetuximab has been shown to alter multiple aspects of antitumor immunity in HNSCC.[43] Thus, the prevailing theory is that cetuximab acts primarily by enhancing antitumor immunity in HNSCC, rather than inhibiting EGFR.[43,44]

Monoclonal antibodies inhibiting immune checkpoints have revolutionized treatment of a variety of cancers, including HNSCC. The cells primarily responsible for killing cancerous cells are cytotoxic T lymphocytes (CTLs). The physiologic purpose of immune checkpoints is to avoid exaggerated immune responses or autoimmunity; however, cancer cells often exploit these molecular targets to avoid CTL killing. The most widely studied of these checkpoints is programmed cell death 1 (PD-1), which binds to its ligand (PD-L1) on cancer cells or other immune cells, thereby dampening the T-cell response (**Fig. 2**). Two monoclonal antibodies blocking PD-1 (pembrolizumab and nivolumab) have been FDA approved for the treatment of recurrent/metastatic HNSCC,[45–47] and there are multiple ongoing clinical trials using checkpoint inhibitors for previously untreated, locally advanced HNSCC.

Another strategy used to enhance the immune response to head and neck cancer is adoptive cell therapy, which consists of infusing T cells or other immune cells into patients who have cancer. Early studies using these techniques for HNSCC have involved collecting the tumor-infiltrating lymphocytes from a tumor, expanding them ex vivo and then reinfusing them into the patient.[48] The success of adoptive T-cell transfer has recently been improved by modifying the T cells to respond to specific antigenic targets. For example, T cells modified to express a receptor specific for the E7 human papillomavirus (HPV) oncoprotein have been used to treat HPV-related HNSCC at the National Cancer Institute (NCT02858310). Engineered chimeric antigen receptor T cells are also under study in HNSCC.[49] Other strategies to enhance immune responses in HNSCC and recurrent respiratory papillomatosis are discussed elsewhere in this issue.

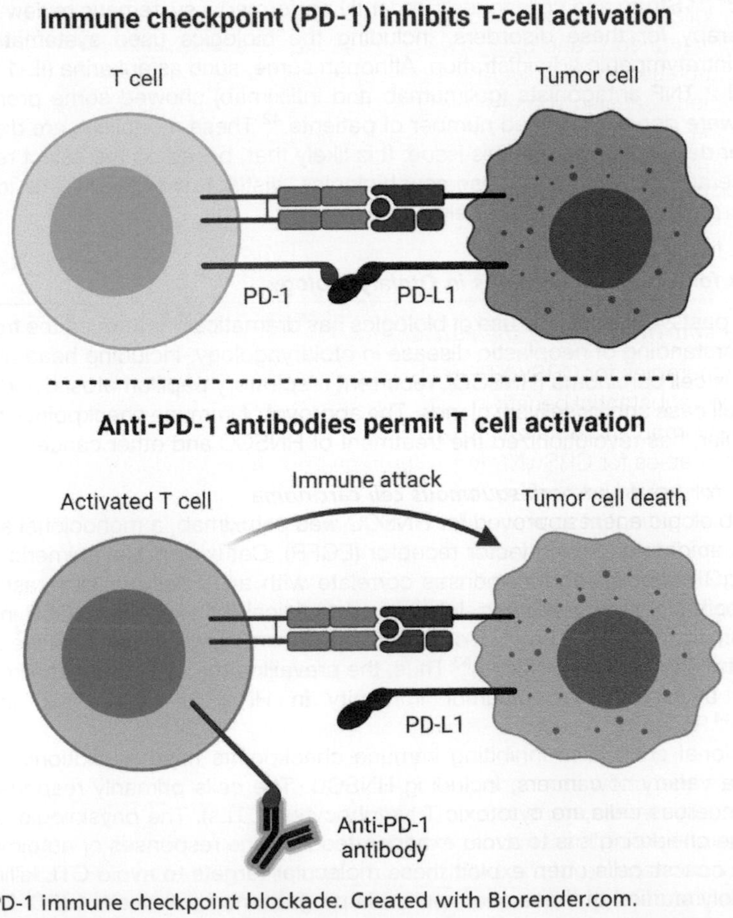

Fig. 2. PD-1 immune checkpoint blockade. Created with Biorender.com.

Biologics for salivary and skull base tumors

Benign and malignant salivary neoplasms are a rare and diverse group of tumors. Genomic studies performed over the past decade have dramatically improved the understanding of salivary tumors and have identified several druggable targets. Salivary duct carcinoma (SDC), an aggressive salivary malignancy, expresses androgen receptor and may respond to androgen deprivation therapy.[50] In other cases of SDC where HER2 is overexpressed, trastuzumab and pertuzumab have been used with remarkable responses.[51] Secretory carcinoma, characterized by an *ETV6–NTRK3* chromosomal fusion, responds very well to the Trk inhibitors larotrectinib and entrectinib.[52] Adenoid cystic carcinoma (ACC) is also characterized by a gene fusion product (MYB-NFIB), but attempts to find a targeted agent that can reliably alter the course of ACC have been disappointing.[52] Salivary malignancies are expected to respond poorly to immune checkpoint blockade because of their low mutational burden; however, some high-grade malignancies that tend to express PD-L1 (eg, SDC) may deserve further study.[53]

Another area where biologics are creating novel treatment options for benign head and neck tumors is in the management of neurofibromatosis type II (NF2). This condition arises from mutation in the gene coding for the Merlin protein, also known as neurofibromin 2 or schwannomin. Because Merlin interacts with multiple intracellular pathways, loss or disfunction of this protein leads to a spectrum of phenotypes, including bilateral vestibular schwannomas, meningiomas, spinal schwannomas, along with cutaneous and ophthalmologic findings.[54] Until recently, surgery and stereotactic radiation therapy were the only treatment options for patients with aggressive mutations causing bilateral vestibular schwannomas. Over the past 2 decades, many of the downstream pathways of the Merlin protein have become targeted for treatment using biologics.[55–58] At present, the biologic with the longest track record is bevacizumab, which was initially used under compassionate care but is now regarded as a favorable treatment option for certain patients with NF2.[59] Treatments available for NF2 and other skull base disorders are further discussed elsewhere in this issue.

Summary and Thoughts for the Future

Targeted therapies for CRSwNP and the family of Th2-mediated respiratory diseases have shown substantial benefit in subjective and objective disease measures. In addition to dupilumab and omalizumab, it is likely that there will be approval for additional biologic therapies for CRSwNP in the future. As experience is gained with these therapies, an improved understanding of disease endotypes and immunologic markers predictive of patient response will play an increasing role in the ability to determine the best candidates for individual biologic therapies. In addition, given the high cost of biologic therapies, cost-benefit analyses will likely play a role in assessment of overall treatment plans. In addition, determination of length of therapy remains a common question in the minds of treating practitioners. Current evidence indicates that biologic therapy for CRSwNP should continue as maintenance therapy, although long-term treatment analyses are lacking at this time (see Roland and Levy's article, "Knowledge Gaps and Research Needs for Biologic Therapy in the Rhinology Practice," in this issue).

Biologics also show immense promise in management of otologic conditions such as chronic otitis media, nonsurgical treatment of tympanic membrane perforation, and sensorineural hearing loss. Furthermore, response to certain biologics should provide a better understanding of the pathophysiology of other conditions, such as autoimmune ear disorders, that are poorly understood at this time.

The future is bright based on the expanding use of biologics to enhance antitumor immunity or to target specific pathways in HNSCC, salivary tumors, and other neoplastic diseases of the head and neck. Although only a minority of patients with recurrent or metastatic disease respond to these agents when used as monotherapy, the use of biologics earlier in the course of the disease and/or in combination with other therapies holds tremendous promise. There are numerous trials underway that are designed to identify biomarkers of response and optimal combinations of immune therapies, targeted therapies, and/or the standard therapies, including surgery, radiation, and cytotoxic chemotherapy.

DISCLOSURE

S.K. Wise: consultant for NeurENT, Stryker; advisory board for OptiNose, SinopSys Surgical, ALK-Abello, and Genentech. N.C. Schmitt: advisory board for Checkpoint Surgical; book royalties from Plural Publishing. A. Monfared: none.

REFERENCES

1. Bren L. The road to the biotech revolution: highlights of 100 years of biologics regulation. Centennial Edition. FDA Consumer; 2006.
2. Lewiecki EM. Biological therapy: chronicling 15 years of progress. Expert Opin Biol Ther 2015;15(5):619–21.
3. Hohl TM. Cell-mediated defense against infection. In: Bennett, Dolin, Blaser, editors. Principles and practice of infectious diseases. 8th edition. Philadelphia: Elsevier; 2015. p. 50–69.
4. Bonecchi R, Sozzani S, Stine JT, et al. Divergent effects of interleukin-4 and interferon-gamma on macrophage-derived chemokine production: an amplification circuit of polarized T helper 2 responses. Blood 1998;92(8):2668–71.
5. Greenfeder S, Umland SP, Cuss FM, et al. Th2 cytokines and asthma. The role of interleukin-5 in allergic eosinophilic disease. Respir Res 2001;2(2):71–9.
6. Kita H. Eosinophils: multifaceted biological properties and roles in health and disease. Immunol Rev 2011;242(1):161–77.
7. McBrien CN, Menzies-Gow A. The biology of eosinophils and their role in asthma. Front Med (Lausanne) 2017;4:93.
8. Bassiouni A, Naidoo Y, Wormald PJ. When FESS fails: the inflammatory load hypothesis in refractory chronic rhinosinusitis. Laryngoscope 2012;122(2):460–6.
9. Gelardi M, Iannuzzi L, De Giosa M, et al. Non-surgical management of chronic rhinosinusitis with nasal polyps based on clinical-cytological grading: a precision medicine-based approach. Acta Otorhinolaryngol Ital 2017;37(1):38–45.
10. Uhliarova B, Kopincova J, Kolomaznik M, et al. Comorbidity has no impact on eosinophil inflammation in the upper airways or on severity of the sinonasal disease in patients with nasal polyps. Clin Otolaryngol 2015;40(5):429–36.
11. Vlaminck S, Vauterin T, Hellings PW, et al. The importance of local eosinophilia in the surgical outcome of chronic rhinosinusitis: a 3-year prospective observational study. Am J Rhinol Allergy 2014;28(3):260–4.
12. Casale TB, Condemi J, LaForce C, et al. Effect of omalizumab on symptoms of seasonal allergic rhinitis: a randomized controlled trial. JAMA 2001;286(23):2956–67.
13. Adelroth E, Rak S, Haahtela T, et al. Recombinant humanized mAb-E25, an anti-IgE mAb, in birch pollen-induced seasonal allergic rhinitis. J Allergy Clin Immunol 2000;106(2):253–9.

14. Okubo K, Ogino S, Nagakura T, et al. Omalizumab is effective and safe in the treatment of Japanese cedar pollen-induced seasonal allergic rhinitis. Allergol Int 2006;55(4):379–86.
15. Chervinsky P, Casale T, Townley R, et al. Omalizumab, an anti-IgE antibody, in the treatment of adults and adolescents with perennial allergic rhinitis. Ann Allergy Asthma Immunol 2003;91(2):160–7.
16. Tsabouri S, Tseretopoulou X, Priftis K, et al. Omalizumab for the treatment of inadequately controlled allergic rhinitis: a systematic review and meta-analysis of randomized clinical trials. J Allergy Clin Immunol Pract 2014;2(3):332–340 e331.
17. Kopp MV, Hamelmann E, Zielen S, et al. Combination of omalizumab and specific immunotherapy is superior to immunotherapy in patients with seasonal allergic rhinoconjunctivitis and co-morbid seasonal allergic asthma. Clin Exp Allergy 2009;39(2):271–9.
18. Kuehr J, Brauburger J, Zielen S, et al. Efficacy of combination treatment with anti-IgE plus specific immunotherapy in polysensitized children and adolescents with seasonal allergic rhinitis. J Allergy Clin Immunol 2002;109(2):274–80.
19. Rolinck-Werninghaus C, Hamelmann E, Keil T, et al. The co-seasonal application of anti-IgE after preseasonal specific immunotherapy decreases ocular and nasal symptom scores and rescue medication use in grass pollen allergic children. Allergy 2004;59(9):973–9.
20. Gevaert P, Omachi TA, Corren J, et al. Efficacy and safety of omalizumab in nasal polyposis: 2 randomized phase 3 trials. J Allergy Clin Immunol 2020;146(3): 595–605.
21. Gevaert P, Van Bruaene N, Cattaert T, et al. Mepolizumab, a humanized anti-IL-5 mAb, as a treatment option for severe nasal polyposis. J Allergy Clin Immunol 2011;128(5):989 95, e981-988.
22. Bachert C, Sousa AR, Lund VJ, et al. Reduced need for surgery in severe nasal polyposis with mepolizumab: Randomized trial. J Allergy Clin Immunol 2017; 140(4):1024–1031 e1014.
23. SYNAPSE media release. 2020. Available at: https://www.gsk.com/en-gb/media/press-releases/nucala-mepolizumab-is-the-first-anti-il5-biologic-to-report-positive-phase-3-results-in-patients-with-nasal-polyps/. Accessed November 4, 2020.
24. Weinstein SF, Katial RK, Bardin P, et al. Effects of reslizumab on asthma outcomes in a subgroup of eosinophilic asthma patients with self-reported chronic rhinosinusitis with nasal polyps. J Allergy Clin Immunol Pract 2019;7(2):589–596 e583.
25. Lombardo N, Pelaia C, Ciriolo M, et al. Real-life effects of benralizumab on allergic chronic rhinosinusitis and nasal polyposis associated with severe asthma. Int J Immunopathol Pharmacol 2020;34. 2058738420950851.
26. Maspero J, Harrison T, Werkstrom V, et al. Clinical efficacy of benralizumab in patients with severe, uncontrolled eosinophilic asthma and nasal polyposis: pooled analysis of the SIROCCO and CALIMA trials. J Allergy Clin Immunol 2018;141: AB12.
27. OSTRO media release. 2020. Available at: https://www.astrazeneca.com/media-centre/press-releases/2020/fasenra-met-both-co-primary-endpoints-of-reduced-nasal-polyp-size-and-blockage-in-the-ostro-phase-iii-trial.html. Accessed November 4, 2020.
28. Bachert C, Han JK, Desrosiers M, et al. Efficacy and safety of dupilumab in patients with severe chronic rhinosinusitis with nasal polyps (LIBERTY NP SINUS-24 and LIBERTY NP SINUS-52): results from two multicentre, randomised, double-blind, placebo-controlled, parallel-group phase 3 trials. Lancet 2019; 394(10209):1638–50.

29. Mudry A. History of myringoplasty and tympanoplasty type I. Otolaryngol Head Neck Surg 2008;139(5):613–4.
30. Jackler RK. A regenerative method of tympanic membrane repair could be the greatest advance in otology since the cochlear implant. Otol Neurotol 2012; 33(3):289.
31. Huang J, Teh BM, Eikelboom RH, et al. The effectiveness of bFGF in the treatment of tympanic membrane perforations: a systematic review and meta-analysis. Otol Neurotol 2020;41(6):782–90.
32. Amoils CP, Jackler RK, Lustig LR. Repair of chronic tympanic membrane perforations using epidermal growth factor. Otolaryngol Head Neck Surg 1992; 107(5):669–83.
33. Lou ZC, Lou Z. Efficacy of EGF and gelatin sponge for traumatic tympanic membrane perforations: a randomized controlled study. Otolaryngol Head Neck Surg 2018;159(6):1028–36.
34. Santa Maria PL, Gottlieb P, Santa Maria C, et al. Functional outcomes of heparin-binding epidermal growth factor-like growth factor for regeneration of chronic tympanic membrane perforations in mice. Tissue Eng Part A 2017;23(9–10): 436–44.
35. Hoffman HJ, Dobie RA, Losonczy KG, et al. Declining prevalence of hearing loss in US adults aged 20 to 69 years. JAMA Otolaryngol Head Neck Surg 2017; 143(3):274–85.
36. WHO. Deafness and hearing loss fact sheet. 2018. Available at: https://www.who.int/news-room/fact-sheets/detail/deafness-and-hearing-loss. Accessed April 1, 2021.
37. Schilder AGM, Su MP, Blackshaw H, et al. Hearing protection, restoration, and regeneration: an overview of emerging therapeutics for inner ear and central hearing disorders. Otol Neurotol 2019;40(5):559–70.
38. Roland JT. Autoimmune inner ear disease. Curr Rheumatol Rep 2000;2(2):171–4.
39. Goodall AF, Siddiq MA. Current understanding of the pathogenesis of autoimmune inner ear disease: a review. Clin Otolaryngol 2015;40(5):412–9.
40. Vambutas A, Pathak S. AAO: autoimmune and autoinflammatory (disease) in otology: what is new in immune-mediated hearing loss. Laryngoscope Investig Otolaryngol 2016;1(5):110–5.
41. Woolf NK, Harris JP. Cochlear pathophysiology associated with inner ear immune responses. Acta Otolaryngol 1986;102(5–6):353–64.
42. Strum D, Kim S, Shim T, et al. An update on autoimmune inner ear disease: a systematic review of pharmacotherapy. Am J Otolaryngol 2020;41(1):102310.
43. Trivedi S, Concha-Benavente F, Srivastava RM, et al. Immune biomarkers of anti-EGFR monoclonal antibody therapy. Ann Oncol 2015;26(1):40–7.
44. Ferris RL, Geiger JL, Trivedi S, et al. Phase II trial of post-operative radiotherapy with concurrent cisplatin plus panitumumab in patients with high-risk, resected head and neck cancer. Ann Oncol 2016;27(12):2257–62.
45. Burtness B, Harrington KJ, Greil R, et al. Pembrolizumab alone or with chemotherapy versus cetuximab with chemotherapy for recurrent or metastatic squamous cell carcinoma of the head and neck (KEYNOTE-048): a randomised, open-label, phase 3 study. The Lancet 2019;394(10212):1915–28.
46. Chow LQM, Haddad R, Gupta S, et al. Antitumor activity of pembrolizumab in biomarker-unselected patients with recurrent and/or metastatic head and neck squamous cell carcinoma: results from the phase Ib KEYNOTE-012 expansion cohort. J Clin Oncol 2016;34(32):3838–45.

47. Ferris RL, Blumenschein G Jr, Fayette J, et al. Nivolumab for recurrent squamous-cell carcinoma of the head and neck. N Engl J Med 2016;375(19):1856–67.
48. Stevanovic S, Helman SR, Wunderlich JR, et al. A phase II study of tumor-infiltrating lymphocyte therapy for human papillomavirus-associated epithelial cancers. Clin Cancer Res 2019;25(5):1486–93.
49. van Schalkwyk MC, Papa SE, Jeannon JP, et al. Design of a phase I clinical trial to evaluate intratumoral delivery of ErbB-targeted chimeric antigen receptor T-cells in locally advanced or recurrent head and neck cancer. Hum Gene Ther Clin Dev 2013;24(3):134–42.
50. Dalin MG, Desrichard A, Katabi N, et al. Comprehensive molecular characterization of salivary duct carcinoma reveals actionable targets and similarity to apocrine breast cancer. Clin Cancer Res 2016;22(18):4623–33.
51. Park JC, Ma TM, Rooper L, et al. Exceptional responses to pertuzumab, trastuzumab, and docetaxel in human epidermal growth factor receptor-2 high expressing salivary duct carcinomas. Head Neck 2018;40(12):E100–6.
52. Di Villeneuve L, Souza IL, Tolentino FDS, et al. Salivary gland carcinoma: novel targets to overcome treatment resistance in advanced disease. Front Oncol 2020;10:580141.
53. Schmitt NC, Kang H, Sharma A. Salivary duct carcinoma: an aggressive salivary gland malignancy with opportunities for targeted therapy. Oral Oncol 2017;74:40–8.
54. Asthagiri AR, Parry DM, Butman JA, et al. Neurofibromatosis type 2. Lancet 2009;373(9679):1974–86.
55. Karajannis MA, Legault G, Hagiwara M, et al. Phase II trial of lapatinib in adult and pediatric patients with neurofibromatosis type 2 and progressive vestibular schwannomas. Neuro Oncol 2012;14(9):1163–70.
56. Sagers JE, Beauchamp RL, Zhang Y, et al. Combination therapy with mTOR kinase inhibitor and dasatinib as a novel therapeutic strategy for vestibular schwannoma. Sci Rep 2020;10(1):4211.
57. Guerrant W, Kota S, Troutman S, et al. YAP mediates tumorigenesis in neurofibromatosis type 2 by promoting cell survival and proliferation through a COX-2-EGFR signaling axis. Cancer Res 2016;76(12):3507–19.
58. Fuse MA, Dinh CT, Vitte J, et al. Preclinical assessment of MEK1/2 inhibitors for neurofibromatosis type 2-associated schwannomas reveals differences in efficacy and drug resistance development. Neuro Oncol 2019;21(4):486–97.
59. Lu VM, Ravindran K, Graffeo CS, et al. Efficacy and safety of bevacizumab for vestibular schwannoma in neurofibromatosis type 2: a systematic review and meta-analysis of treatment outcomes. J Neurooncol 2019;144(2):239–48.

Current Evidence for Biologic Therapy in Chronic Rhinosinusitis with Nasal Polyposis

Uma S. Ramaswamy, MD, Katie Melder, MD, Vijay A. Patel, MD, Stella E. Lee, MD*

KEYWORDS

• Biologics • Chronic rhinosinusitis • Monoclonal antibody • Nasal polyposis

KEY POINTS

- Current evidence suggests biologic therapy for chronic rhinosinusitis with nasal polyps (CRSwNP) leads to decreased polyp burden and improvement in quality of life by selectively blocking type 2 inflammatory pathways.
- Dupilumab, which blocks interleukin (IL)-4 and IL-13, and omalizumab, which binds free immunoglobulin E, are monoclonal antibodies that are currently approved by the US Food and Drug Administration for treatment of uncontrolled CRSwNP.
- Mepolizumab, which binds free IL-5, and benralizumab, which blocks the IL-5 receptor, have also been investigated for the treatment of CRSwNP, and results from the phase III trials are pending.
- Other therapeutics in the pipeline include tezepepelumab, which binds thymic stromal lymphopoietin, and fevipiprant, an antagonist of the prostaglandin D_2 receptor 2.

INTRODUCTION

The problem surrounding the management of chronic rhinosinusitis with nasal polyposis (CRSwNP) has captivated practitioners for over 2 millennia. Derived from the Greek word πωλυποζ (pôlupos), meaning many feet, like an octopus, Hippocrates was among the first physicians to describe nasal polyposis and propose remedies including topical honey, iron cauterization, and snare polypectomy in his fabled text *Diseases II*.[1] As understanding of CRSwNP pathophysiology expanded over time, modern treatment principles revolved around topical medications including intranasal

Department of Otolaryngology–Head and Neck Surgery, University of Pittsburgh Medical Center, 1400 Locust Street, Suite 2100, Pittsburgh, PA 15219, USA
* Corresponding author. Department of Otolaryngology–Head and Neck Surgery, Division of Sinonasal Disorders and Allergy, University of Pittsburgh Medical Center, 1400 Locust Street, Suite 2100, Pittsburgh, PA 15219.
E-mail address: stellaeunlee@gmail.com

Otolaryngol Clin N Am 54 (2021) 689–699
https://doi.org/10.1016/j.otc.2021.04.007
0030-6665/21/

corticosteroids and saline irrigations, as well as systemic drugs such as oral corticosteroids and antimicrobials for symptomatic flares. In cases of failure of appropriate medical therapy, functional endoscopic sinus surgery (FESS) allows for the restoration of paranasal sinus patency, removal of obstructive polypoid tissue, and improved access for topical medication delivery to the sinuses.[2] Although this current paradigm is effective for most individuals with CRSwNP, there remains a subset of patients with recalcitrant disease that is difficult to control. Risk factors for polyp recurrence include allergic fungal rhinosinusitis, aspirin-exacerbated respiratory disease (AERD), comorbid asthma, and prior polypectomy.[3] The manifestations of CRSwNP extend beyond the nose and paranasal sinuses, as it carries a significant impact on quality-of-life (QOL). Patients with CRSwNP experience cognitive impairment and depression, as well as overall health state utility values equal to or worse than other chronic health ailments such as congestive heart failure, chronic obstructive pulmonary disease, and end-stage renal disease.[4–6]

The financial implications of CRSwNP are also substantial, with annual incremental costs $11,507 higher compared to those without chronic rhinosinusitis and a total national economic burden of $22 billion (direct and indirect costs) in 2014.[7,8] With the advent of biologic agents, targeted disease and cell-specific therapy have become available for various immune-mediated conditions including asthma, atopic dermatitis, and urticaria.[9–11] These treatments derive their utility by directly intervening in dysfunctional immune pathways, and many of the therapeutics trialed in CRSwNP have their origins in asthma treatment.[12] Although there is significant overlap between these diseases, it is interesting that some biologic agents that are effective in asthma may not be as effective in CRS, demonstrating that although the upper and lower airways are unified in some ways, there are distinct differences in disease pathophysiology and treatment response that should be considered.

PATHOPHYSIOLOGY

As understanding of CRS continues to expand beyond the presence or absence of nasal polyposis, a greater appreciation of disease endotypes has allowed for improved characterization of disease patterns with the added ability to allow for a more personalized and efficacious treatment regimen. Recent research efforts focused on CRSwNP endotyping have revealed mixed profiles sustained by several inflammatory signatures, which vary according to ethnicity and geographic region. Further research using advanced techniques in single-cell mRNA sequencing has revealed the diversity of cell types and molecular pathways that may be contributing to the pathophysiology of disease.[13]

Type 1 inflammation is sustained by T_H1 polarization with prevalent neutrophilic infiltration and interferon (IFN)-γ overproduction; this endotype is most common in East Asian (China) individuals with CRSwNP.[14] Conversely, most Caucasian (North American and European) patients (80%–85%) with CRSwNP present with type 2 inflammation, defined by a predominance of interleukin (IL)-4, IL-5, and IL-13, with a sinonasal infiltrate rich in eosinophils, mast cells, and T_H2 cells. Although sinonasal epithelia serve as the first line of innate defense in the upper airway, they express multiple pattern recognition receptors to sense and react to proteolytic allergens, harmful microbes, particulates, and tissue injury, which can trigger type 2 inflammation.[15]

In CRSwNP, sinonasal mucosa or solitary chemosensory cells produce IL-1, IL-25, IL-33, and TSLP in response to molecular patterns (ATP and HMGB), micro-organisms (*Staphylococcus aureus* and fungi), pathogenic byproducts (microbial DNA and toxins), and/or allergens.[16–18] The production of IL-33 and TSLP leads to type 2 innate lymphocyte activation, with subsequent production of IL-5 and IL-13.[19] IL-13 drives immunoglobulin E (IgE) class switching in B cells, leading to elevated local IgE, a known feature of nasal polypsosis.[20] Additionally, IL-13 leads to endothelial vascular cell adhesion protein 1 expression, enabling lymphocyte, eosinophil, and basophil recruitment.[20] IL-13 also drives recruited monocyte differentiation to alternatively activated macrophages, a phenotype with impaired phagocytosis that is known to accumulate in nasal polyposis.[21] IL-5 plays a key role in stimulating eosinophil activation, growth, recruitment, and survival.[22] This cycle of type 2 inflammation results in increased vascular permeability and toxic eosinophil protein release, inducing epithelial erosion, impaired ciliary function, and mucus hypersecretion, which sets the stage for inflammatory polyposis.[23]

Finally, type 3 inflammation is characterized by increased release of IL-17 with a mixed inflammatory cell pattern including involvement of neutrophils, mast cells, T_H17, and T_H22 cells.[24] Although challenging, defining a patient's endotype will be important in the future. By identifying specific immunologic processes involved in CRSwNP one can be better informed on optimal therapeutic strategies that are tailored to the particular variant of disease.

CLINICAL TRIALS OF BIOLOGICS FOR NASAL POLYPOSIS

Patients with CRSwNP have traditionally been treated with a combination of nasal irrigations, intranasal and oral corticosteroids, sinus surgery, and oral and/or topical antibiotics during exacerbations. Although surgery may initially be successful, studies have shown a significant relapse, 20% at 1 year and 80% at 12 years, despite consistent intranasal corticosteroid treatment.[25] Recent clinical trials studying biologic agents in the management of CRSwNP, however, offer patients and clinicians with additional treatment options that may help avoid the potential complications and adverse effects of systemic corticosteroid therapy and multiple sinus surgeries.[26,27]

TARGETING INTERLEUKIN-4 AND INTERLEUKIN-13

Dupilumab

Dupilumab is a fully human monoclonal antibody that inhibits IL-4 and IL-13 signaling by blocking the alpha subunit of the IL-4 receptor. Dupilumab was approved by the US Food and Drug Administration (FDA) in June 2019 for the treatment of adult CRSwNP patients with inadequately controlled disease. The first trial investigating dupilumab for CRSwNP was conducted from 2013 to 2014 with 60 patients randomized to dupilumab 600 mg loading dose followed by 15 weekly doses of 300 mg (n = 30) or placebo (n = 30) for 16 weeks.[28] These patients had CRSwNP refractory to intranasal corticosteroids and were eligible if they demonstrated a mean nasal polyp score (NPS) of 5 (out of a maximum of 8), a minimum score of 2 for each nostril and symptoms of uncontrolled CRS. The primary end point was mean change in NPS from baseline to week 16. Secondary end points included Lund-Mackay score (LMS), Sinonasal Outcome Test (SNOT)-22, University of Pennsylvania Smell Identification Test (UPSIT) score, and peak nasal inspiratory flow (PNIF). Asthma outcomes were also measured, as well as total serum IgE, blood eosinophils, serum thymus and activation regulated chemokine (TARC) level, and eotaxin-3 plasma level. Dupilumab was effective in decreasing polyp size, with a mean difference between groups of NPS = −1.6 (P<.001). Significant improvements were also seen for LMS (mean group difference −8.8), SNOT-22 (mean group difference −18.1), and UPSIT (mean group difference 14.8), all favoring dupilumab treatment. In addition, reductions in IgE, TARC, and eotaxin-3 were noted with dupilumab treatment. There was an increase in blood eosinophil counts at week 4, but by week 16, the mean counts were unchanged. No serious adverse events were reported related to dupilumab therapy.

Two phase 3 trials followed, LIBERTY NP SINUS-24 and LIBERTY NP SINUS-52, evaluating the efficacy of dupilumab in poorly controlled CRSwNP in a larger study population (**Table 1**).[29] Patients were similarly enrolled if they fulfilled criteria for severe disease including NPS of at least 5, a nasal congestion score (NCS) of at least 2 out of a maximum of 3 (0 = asymptomatic, 1 = mild, 2 = moderate, and 3 = severe), and had received oral corticosteroids (OCS) in the preceding 2 years or had undergone sinus surgery previously. In both SINUS-24 and SINUS-52, short-course OCS and sinus surgery were permitted. Patients underwent a 4-week run-in period during which patients were maintained on topical 100 μg of mometasone furoate nasal spray in each nostril twice daily. Patients were then randomized to either 300 mg of dupilumab subcutaneously or placebo every 2 weeks for 24 weeks in the SINUS-24 trial or in one of 3 groups for 52 weeks in SINUS-52: dupilumab every 2 weeks, placebo, or every 2 weeks for 24 weeks and then every 4 weeks for the remaining 28 weeks. Patients were followed for an additional 24 weeks in SINUS-24 and an additional 12 weeks in SINUS-52.

Coprimary endpoints for both trials were change in NPS and NCS at week 24. Key secondary endpoints were change in UPSIT, SNOT-22, LMS, total symptom score, and daily loss of smell score. Blood biomarkers including eosinophil count, serum total IgE, TARC, periostin, and plasma eotaxin-3 were obtained. Nasal secretions were analyzed for eosinophil cationic protein (ECP), eotaxin-3, and total IgE.

In SINUS-24, 143 patients were randomized to dupilumab, and 133 patients were randomized to placebo. In SINUS 52, 150 patients were randomized to dupilumab every 2 weeks; 145 patients were randomized to dupilumab every 2 weeks until week 24 and then every 4 weeks, and 153 patients were randomized to placebo. In the total study population, more than half of patients had asthma (n = 428, 59%); about a quarter had AERD (n = 204, 28%). Most patients had undergone surgery (n = 459, 63% with ≥1 surgery and n = 111, 15% with ≥3 surgeries), and most were treated with OCS in the preceding 2 years (n = 538, 74%). Patients had an average NPS of 5.97 and anosmia at baseline (n = 551, 76%).

Dupilumab was effective in decreasing polyp size and improving quality of life, most notably with the return of smell. At 24 weeks, the mean difference between groups was an improvement in NPS of −2.06 in SINUS-24 and -1.80 in SINUS-52. Patients also had improvements in NCS, SNOT-22, LMS, and UPSIT (see **Table 1**). Hazard ratios demonstrated a 74% reduction for OCS need in the dupilumab group compared with placebo and an 83% reduction in the need for sinus surgery with dupilumab treatment. Overall dupilumab was well tolerated, but 4 cases of eosinophilic granulomatosis with polyangiitis (EGPA) were reported, three of which occurred in the dupilumab group, and one in the placebo group. This is an area that warrants further study, as patients with type 2 inflammation often present with elevated levels of eosinophils and may be at risk for possible EGPA.

TARGETING IMMUNOGLOBULIN E

Omalizumab

One of the first monoclonal antibodies to be approved for use was omalizumab. Omalizumab is a DNA-derived humanized IgG1 monoclonal antibody that binds free IgE, preventing its interaction with the FcεRI receptor on mast cells and basophils. It also reduces the expression of this high-affinity receptor on mast cells, basophils, and dendritic cells. It decreases T_H2-cell activation and proliferation by decreasing mast cell degranulation, thereby blocking the release of mast-cell derived cytokines

Table 1
Summary of phase 3 clinical trial data

	Omalizumab	Mepolizumab	Dupilumab
Clinical trial	POLYP 1 and POLYP 2	SYNAPSE	SINUS-24 and SINUS-52
Target pathway	IgE	IL-5	IL-4/IL-13
Mechanism of action	Monoclonal antibody anti-IgE	Monoclonal antibody anti-IL-5	Monoclonal antibody anti-IL-4Rα
Study population	Adults with ICS-refractory CRSwNP: POLYP 1 (n = 138) POLYP 2 (n = 127) AERD n = 72 (27%)	Adults with previous surgery and/or need for further (n = 407); AERD n = 108 (26.5%)	Adults with bilateral CRSwNP refractory to ICS, receiving OCS within 2 y or surgery (n = 724); AERD n = 204 (28%)
Time point	24 weeks	52 weeks	24 and 52 weeks
Administration and dosage	SC injection of 75–600 mg omalizumab vs placebo (both groups received background intranasal mometasone), dosed every 2–4 weeks (based on patient weight and IgE levels) for 24 weeks	SC injection of 100 mg mepolizumab vs placebo, dosed every 4 weeks for 52 weeks	SINUS-24: SC injection of 300 mg dupilumab vs placebo, dosed every 2 weeks for 24 weeks SINUS-52: SC injection of 300 mg dupilumab every 2 weeks for 52 weeks vs SC 300 mg dupilumab every 2 weeks for 24 weeks then every 4 weeks for an additional 28 weeks vs placebo
Change in NPS	−1.14, −0.59	−0.73 (median)	−2.06, −1.80
NCS	−0.55, −0.50		−0.89, −0.87
Nasal obstruction (VAS)	N/A	−3.14	N/A
SNOT-22	-16.12, -15.04	−16.5 (median)	−21.12, −17.36
UPSIT	3.81, 3.86	N/A	10.56, 10.52
Lund-Mackay CT score	N/A	N/A	-7.44, -5.13
Need for SCS	62.5% reduction (*P*=.16)	Odds ratio to placebo (95% CI): 0.58 (0.36, 0.92) *P*=.020	73.9% reduction
Need for surgery	Odds ratio 6.3, 6.2	57% reduction	83% reduction

and their effects on B and T cells and eosinophils, suppressing the body's inflammatory response.[15]

For over a decade, this drug has been successfully used in patients with severe asthma.[10,30,31] In 2013, the FDA also approved the use of omalizumab in patients with chronic urticaria.[9,32,33] Early case reports and small, uncontrolled studies purported some benefit in asthma patients with concomitant nasal polyps.[15] Bidder and colleagues[34] conducted a real-life study in 2018, concluding that omalizumab improves comorbid CRSwNP in patients with severe asthma.

In 2004, Pinto and colleagues performed a randomized, double-blind, placebo-controlled trial of omalizumab for the treatment of CRS patients with and without nasal polyps. The primary outcome was quantitative measure of inflammation on maxillofacial computed tomography (CT) scans. Secondary outcomes included cellular inflammation, QOL and symptom scores (SNOT-20), nasal airflow (NPIF), and olfaction (UPSIT). Although inflammation was reduced on imaging in patients treated with omalizumab, the net difference after treatment between both arms was not significant. SNOT-20 scores at 3, 5, and 6 months did improve in those patients treated with omalizumab, but all other measures showed no difference between placebo and treatment groups. The negative results of this pilot study, however, could be secondary to small sample size (14 patients) and the mixed cohort of CRSsNP and CRSwNP patients. They concluded that while IgE does seem to be involved with the inflammatory response and symptomatology in patients with CRS, larger studies would be necessary to prove any clinically significant benefit.[35,36]

On Dec. 1, 2020, the FDA approved omalizumab for use in adults with CRSwNP based on results of the POLYP 1 and POLYP 2 trials. These were replicate, phase 3, randomized, double-blind, multicenter, placebo-controlled studies that evaluated the safety and efficacy of omalizumab in adult CRSwNP patients with inadequate response to intranasal corticosteroids. Coprimary end points included NPS and NCS at the end of the 24-week treatment period (see **Table 1**). Secondary outcomes were SNOT-22, UPSIT, and Asthma Quality of Life Questionnaire (AQLQ) scores in those with concurrent asthma, sense of smell, postnasal drip, rhinorrhea, and adverse events.[15,25]

One hundred thirty-eight and 127 patients were randomized in each study, respectively. Baseline NPS was at least 6, and SNOT-22 scores were at least $\geq$60, consistent with significant disease-related impairment. Both studies showed significant improvement in NPS by at least 1 or 2 points, respectively. Concurrent symptomatic improvement in postnasal drip, rhinorrhea, and sense of smell were also reported. SNOT-22 scores showed significant improvement in QOL in both trials (−24.7 vs −8.6 [P<.0001] and −21.6 vs −6.6 [P<.0001]). Asthma-related QOL also improved in these patients, as demonstrated by at least a 0.5-point improvement in AQLQ scores.[15,25]

The most commonly observed adverse events in these studies included headache, injection site reactions, dizziness, arthralgias, and upper abdominal pain. Contraindications to omalizumab included helminthic infection, cancer, and known allergic reaction to omalizumab or any of its components (see **Table 1**).[15,25]

TARGETING INTERLEUKIN (IL-5)

Mepolizumab

Mepolizumab is an anti-IL-5 monoclonal antibody that binds directly to IL-5, thus preventing receptor binding. Gevaert and colleagues[37] published one of the first studies investigating mepolizumab as a treatment option for severe nasal polyposis (defined as NPS 3 or 4 or recurrence after surgery). This double-blind study randomized 30 patients to receive mepolizumab or placebo (20 and 10 patients, respectively). Mepolizumab was given as two 750 mg intravenous injections 28 days apart. Over half (60%) of the mepolizumab group had a statistically significant reduction in size of nasal polyps at 8 weeks as measured by endoscopic scoring.[37]

In a larger, double-blind, placebo-controlled trial in 2017, Bachert and colleagues[38] randomized 105 patients to receive 750 mg intravenous injections of mepolizumab or placebo every 4 weeks for a total of 6 doses in addition to daily intranasal corticosteroid use. Patients included had CRSwNP recalcitrant to medical therapy (daily intranasal corticosteroids) and were candidates for sinus surgery. The need for surgery was defined as NPS of at least 3 in 1 nostril and a minimum NPS of 2 in the contralateral nostril, as well as a visual analog scale (VAS) score greater than 7. The primary outcome was the need for surgery at the conclusion of the study. The mepolizumab arm had a significantly greater percentage of patients who were no longer deemed surgical candidates at week 25 (30% vs 10%, $P=.006$). The mean SNOT-22 scores were significantly improved in mepolizumab group compared with placebo at week 25 (27.1 vs 40.1, respectively; $P=.005$). In addition, several other secondary end points showed significantly favorable results with mepolizumab such as NP severity, VAS score, and endoscopic NPS. The safety profile of mepolizumab was comparable to placebo (5% vs 3% adverse events, respectively).[38]

The SYNAPSE trial is the largest mepolizumab study to date, and is a double-blind, parallel-group, phase 3 study that[39] randomized 407 patients with prior polyp surgery and/or need for surgery with 100 mg subcutaneous mepolizumab versus placebo, dosed every 4 weeks for 52 weeks. The primary outcomes, endoscopic NPS, and nasal obstruction VAS score were significantly improved with mepolizumab.[40] In addition, this study also showed significantly improved SNOT-22, overall VAS score, and reduced need for surgery in the treatment group.

Reslizumab

Reslizumab is another anti-IL-5 monoclonal antibody; however, there is less evidence regarding its efficacy in CRSwNP. An early phase study by Gevaert and colleagues[22] randomized 24 patients with bilateral nasal polyposis (grade 3/4) or recurrent NP after surgery to single intravenous infusion of 3 mg/kg reslizumab, 1 mg/kg reslizumab, or placebo. The NPS was significantly reduced in a subset of treated patients (50%), who were termed "responders". Interestingly, nasal IL-5 levels predicted which patients would be responders, with levels greater than 40 pg/mL predicting positive response to the drug (odds ratio 21.0, $P=.009$). This phase 1 study demonstrated the safety of a single dose of reslizumab and suggested that this biologic agent may be a good option for patients with high nasal IL-5 levels.[22]

Benralizumab

Benralizumab is an anti-IL-5Rα antibody that works by binding the alpha component of the IL-5 receptor on eosinophils and basophils and thus effectively blocking IL-5 binding. There is an ongoing multicenter phase III trial, OSTRO, which has enrolled 413 patients with CRSwNP recalcitrant to medical and surgical therapy over 56 weeks.[41] These patients were randomized to 30 mg subcutaneous benralizumab or placebo. In addition, both groups received intranasal mometasone. NPS and patient-reported nasal blockage were the primary measurements of this study. Data have not yet been published and are expected in August 2021.

IN THE PIPELINE

Other biologic agents in the pipeline that show promise in treating CRSwNP include tezepelumab and fevipiprant. Tezepelumab is a monoclonal antibody that binds TSLP. TSLP is an upstream cytokine that plays a role in airway hyperresponsiveness and is overexpressed in patients with severe asthma. Preliminary trials show promise for the use of tezepelumab in treating severe asthma.[42] Nagarkar and colleagues[18] showed that TSLP mRNA was not only upregulated in CRSwNP, but also positively correlated with eosinophils and type 2 cytokines, suggesting the clinical relevance of TSLP in the pathophysiology of CRSwNP and the potential value of tezepelumab in treating CRSwNP.

Fevipripant is an oral antagonist of the prostaglandin D_2 receptor 2. Phase 2 trials of fevipripant found that it decreased sputum eosinophils and improved lung function in patients with asthma. Although recent phase 3 trials (LUSTER-1 and LUSTER-2) showed consistent and modest reduction in rates of asthma exacerbations, these results were not statistically significant.[43] Currently, a phase 3, proof-of-concept study is underway to evaluate the ability of fevipripant to reduce NPS in CRSwNP patients with concomitant asthma.[44]

SUMMARY

As our understanding of the pathomechanisms of CRSwNP increases, other targets and pathways will be investigated to treat this condition. It is an exciting time in CRS research, as these biologic trials are also providing new insights into the possible mechanisms of disease and presenting a new paradigm of how CRS is understood and ultimately treated. It is important to realize that these biologic therapies have not yet demonstrated a disease-modifying effect, and symptoms often return once therapy is discontinued. In the future, it is the hope that the underlying drivers of inflammation can be determined in order to prevent and potentially cure CRS.

DISCLOSURE

S.E. Lee has received clinical trial funding and participated on advisory boards for AstraZeneca, Genentech, Genzyme, GlaxoSmithKline, Sanofi-Aventis, and Regeneron.

REFERENCES

1. Mudry A. An octopus in the nostrils. Eur Ann Otorhinolaryngol Head Neck Dis 2020;137(3):211–2.
2. Alobid I, Mullol J. Role of medical therapy in the management of nasal polyps. Curr Allergy Asthma Rep 2012;12(2):144–53.
3. Loftus CA, Soler ZM, Koochakzadeh S, et al. Revision surgery rates in chronic rhinosinusitis with nasal polyps: meta-analysis of risk factors. Int Forum Allergy Rhinol 2020;10(2):199–207.
4. Schlosser RJ, Hyer JM, Smith TL, et al. Depression-specific outcomes after treatment of chronic rhinosinusitis. JAMA Otolaryngol Head Neck Surg 2016;142(4):370–6.
5. Soler ZM, Wittenberg E, Schlosser RJ, et al. Health state utility values in patients undergoing endoscopic sinus surgery. Laryngoscope 2011;121(12):2672–8.
6. Yoo F, Schlosser RJ, Storck KA, et al. Effects of endoscopic sinus surgery on objective and subjective measures of cognitive dysfunction in chronic rhinosinusitis. Int Forum Allergy Rhinol 2019;9(10):1135–43.

7. Bhattacharyya N, Villeneuve S, Joish VN, et al. Cost burden and resource utilization in patients with chronic rhinosinusitis and nasal polyps. Laryngoscope 2019; 129(9):1969–75.
8. Smith KA, Orlandi RR, Rudmik L. Cost of adult chronic rhinosinusitis: a systematic review. Laryngoscope 2015;125(7):1547–56.
9. Asero R. Efficacy of omalizumab 150 mg/month as a maintenance dose in patients with severe chronic spontaneous urticaria showing a prompt and complete response to the drug. Allergy 2018;73(11):2242–4.
10. Busse WW. Anti-immunoglobulin E (omalizumab) therapy in allergic asthma. Am J Respir Crit Care Med 2001;164(8 Pt 2):S12–7.
11. Simpson EL, Akinlade B, Ardeleanu M. Two phase 3 trials of dupilumab versus placebo in atopic dermatitis. N Engl J Med 2017;376(11):1090–1.
12. Willson TJ, Naclerio RM, Lee SE. Monoclonal antibodies for the treatment of nasal polyps. Immunol Allergy Clin North Am 2017;37(2):357–67.
13. Ordovas-Montanes J, Dwyer DF, Nyquist SK, et al. Allergic inflammatory memory in human respiratory epithelial progenitor cells. Nature 2018;560(7720):649–54.
14. Ba L, Zhang N, Meng J, et al. The association between bacterial colonization and inflammatory pattern in Chinese chronic rhinosinusitis patients with nasal polyps. Allergy 2011;66(10):1296–303.
15. Bachert C, Zhang N, Cavaliere C, et al. Biologics for chronic rhinosinusitis with nasal polyps. J Allergy Clin Immunol 2020;145(3):725–39.
16. Kohanski MA, Workman AD, Patel NN, et al. Solitary chemosensory cells are a primary epithelial source of IL-25 in patients with chronic rhinosinusitis with nasal polyps. J Allergy Clin Immunol 2018;142(2):460–9.e7.
17. Lan F, Zhang N, Holtappels G, et al. *Staphylococcus aureus* induces a mucosal type 2 immune response via epithelial cell-derived cytokines. Am J Respir Crit Care Med 2018;198(4):452–63.
18. Nagarkar DR, Poposki JA, Tan BK, et al. Thymic stromal lymphopoietin activity is increased in nasal polyps of patients with chronic rhinosinusitis. J Allergy Clin Immunol 2013;132(3):593–600.e2.
19. Poposki JA, Klingler AI, Tan BK, et al. Group 2 innate lymphoid cells are elevated and activated in chronic rhinosinusitis with nasal polyps. Immun Inflamm Dis 2017;5(3):233–43.
20. Bochner BS, Klunk DA, Sterbinsky SA, et al. IL-13 selectively induces vascular cell adhesion molecule-1 expression in human endothelial cells. J Immunol 1995;154(2):799–803.
21. Krysko O, Holtappels G, Zhang N, et al. Alternatively activated macrophages and impaired phagocytosis of S. aureus in chronic rhinosinusitis. Allergy 2011;66(3): 396–403.
22. Gevaert P, Lang-Loidolt D, Lackner A, et al. Nasal IL-5 levels determine the response to anti-IL-5 treatment in patients with nasal polyps. J Allergy Clin Immunol 2006;118(5):1133–41.
23. Ponikau JU, Winter LA, Kephart GM, et al. An immunologic test for chronic rhinosinusitis based on free intranasal eosinophilic major basic protein. Int Forum Allergy Rhinol 2015;5(1):28–35.
24. Makihara S, Okano M, Fujiwara T, et al. Regulation and characterization of IL-17A expression in patients with chronic rhinosinusitis and its relationship with eosinophilic inflammation. J Allergy Clin Immunol 2010;126(2):397–400, 400.e1-11.
25. Gevaert P, Omachi TA, Corren J, et al. Efficacy and safety of omalizumab in nasal polyposis: 2 randomized phase 3 trials. J Allergy Clin Immunol 2020;146(3): 595–605.

26. Laidlaw TM, Buchheit KM. Biologics in chronic rhinosinusitis with nasal polyposis. Ann Allergy Asthma Immunol 2020;124(4):326–32.
27. Ren L, Zhang N, Zhang L, et al. Biologics for the treatment of chronic rhinosinusitis with nasal polyps - state of the art. World Allergy Organ J 2019;12(8):100050.
28. Bachert C, Mannent L, Naclerio RM, et al. Effect of subcutaneous dupilumab on nasal polyp burden in patients with chronic sinusitis and nasal polyposis: a randomized clinical trial. JAMA 2016;315(5):469–79.
29. Bachert C, Han JK, Desrosiers M, et al. Efficacy and safety of dupilumab in patients with severe chronic rhinosinusitis with nasal polyps (LIBERTY NP SINUS-24 and LIBERTY NP SINUS-52): results from two multicentre, randomised, double-blind, placebo-controlled, parallel-group phase 3 trials. Lancet 2019; 394(10209):1638–50.
30. Ayres JG, Higgins B, Chilvers ER, et al. Efficacy and tolerability of anti-immunoglobulin E therapy with omalizumab in patients with poorly controlled (moderate-to-severe) allergic asthma. Allergy 2004;59(7):701–8.
31. Liebhaber M, Dyer Z. Home therapy with subcutaneous anti-immunoglobulin-E antibody omalizumab in 25 patients with immunoglobulin-E-mediated (allergic) asthma. J Asthma 2007;44(3):195–6.
32. Maurer M, Rosen K, Hsieh HJ, et al. Omalizumab for the treatment of chronic idiopathic or spontaneous urticaria. N Engl J Med 2013;368(10):924–35.
33. Wu KCP, Jabbar-Lopez ZK. Omalizumab, an anti-IgE mAb, receives approval for the treatment of chronic idiopathic/spontaneous urticaria. J Invest Dermatol 2015; 135(1):13–5.
34. Bidder T, Sahota J, Rennie C, et al. Omalizumab treats chronic rhinosinusitis with nasal polyps and asthma together-a real life study. Rhinology 2018;56(1):42–5.
35. Bachert C, Desrosiers MY, Hellings PW, et al. The role of biologics in chronic rhinosinusitis with nasal polyps. J Allergy Clin Immunol Pract 2021;9(3):1099–106.
36. Pinto JM, Mehta N, DiTineo M, et al. A randomized, double-blind, placebo-controlled trial of anti-IgE for chronic rhinosinusitis. Rhinology 2010;48(3):318–24.
37. Gevaert P, Van Bruaene N, Cattaert T, et al. Mepolizumab, a humanized anti-IL-5 mAb, as a treatment option for severe nasal polyposis. J Allergy Clin Immunol 2011;128(5):989–95.e1-8.
38. Bachert C, Sousa AR, Lund VJ, et al. Reduced need for surgery in severe nasal polyposis with mepolizumab: randomized trial. J Allergy Clin Immunol 2017; 140(4):1024–31.e14.
39. Medicine USNLo. A randomised, double-blind, parallel group PhIII study to assess the clinical efficacy and safety of 100 mg SC mepolizumab as an add on to maintenance treatment in adults with severe bilateral nasal polyps - SYNAPSE (StudY in NAsal Polyps Patients to Assess the Safety and Efficacy of Mepolizumab). Available at: ClinicalTrials.gov https://clinicaltrials.gov/ct2/show/NCT03085797?term=mepolizumab+and+nasal+polyps&rank=1. Accessed June 18, 2021.
40. Han JK, Bachert C, Fokkens W, et al. SYNAPSE study investigators. Mepolizumab for chronic rhinosinusitis with nasal polyps (SYNAPSE): a randomised, double-blind, placebo-controlled, phase 3 trial. Lancet Respir Med 2021;16:S2213-2600(21)00097-7. doi: 10.1016/S2213-2600(21)00097-7. Epub ahead of print. PMID: 33872587.
41. Medicine USNLo. A multicenter, randomized, double-blind, parallel-group, placebo-controlled phase 3 efficacy and safety study of benralizumab in patients with severe nasal polyposis. Available at: https://clinicaltrials.gov/ct2/show/

NCT03401229?term=benralizumab&cond=nasal+polyps&draw=2&rank=3. Accessed June 18, 2021.
42. Marone G, Spadaro G, Braile M, et al. Tezepelumab: a novel biological therapy for the treatment of severe uncontrolled asthma. Expert Opin Investig Drugs 2019;28(11):931–40.
43. Brightling CE, Gaga M, Inoue H, et al. Effectiveness of fevipiprant in reducing exacerbations in patients with severe asthma (LUSTER-1 and LUSTER-2): two phase 3 randomised controlled trials. Lancet Respir Med 2021;9(1):43–56.
44. Medicine USNLo. Study of efficacy of fevipiprant in patients with nasal polyposis and asthma (THUNDER). Available at: https://clinicaltrials.gov/ct2/show/NCT03681093?term=fevipiprant+thunder&draw=2&rank=1. https://clinicaltrials.gov/ct2/show/NCT03401229?term=benralizumab&cond=nasal+polyps&draw=2&rank=3. Accessed June 18, 2021.

Choosing the Right Patient for Biologic Therapy in Chronic Rhinosinusitis with Nasal Polyposis

Endotypes, Patient Characteristics, and Defining Failures of Standard Therapy

Michael P. Platt, MD, MSc*, Christopher D. Brook, MD

KEYWORDS

• Sinusitis • Polyps • Biologics • Sinus surgery • Endotypes

KEY POINTS

- Sinusitis research has identified disease endotypes that have distinct clinical behaviors and pathophysiologies, and have allowed for further delineation and characterization for targeted treatments.
- Chronic sinusitis is a spectrum of disease severity and comorbidities requiring a personalized approach to find the best treatment for the appropriate patient.
- Understanding the individual nuances of the different endotypes and characteristics of disease can allow for more precise treatment.
- Endotyping of chronic sinusitis often requires detailed biologic and clinical information, physical examination, radiographic studies, tissue histology, and other adjunct markers of inflammation.
- Biologic treatment for patients with chronic sinusitis with polyps should be considered for patients who have refractory disease despite appropriate medical therapy, and comprehensive surgery, and those who are poor surgical candidates, are surgically averse, or have comorbid conditions such as asthma that may benefit from a biologic agent.

INTRODUCTION

With the advent of any new treatment option for a chronic, complex disease, questions arise regarding the appropriate place where the new therapy fits in a treatment algorithm already containing numerous options. The studies used for regulatory approval

Department of Otolaryngology–Head and Neck Surgery, 800 Harrison Avenue BCD5, Boston, MA 02118, USA
* Corresponding author.
E-mail address: Michael.platt@bmc.org

Otolaryngol Clin N Am 54 (2021) 701–708
https://doi.org/10.1016/j.otc.2021.04.008 oto.theclinics.com

of biologic therapies for nasal polyposis[1,2] did not include any comparative groups with accepted and/or standard clinical treatments. Therefore, expert opinion and clinical decision making will drive recommendations until future studies delineate where monoclonal antibodies or biologic agents fit in clinical treatment algorithms for nasal polyposis. Patients with chronic rhinosinusitis (CRS) with nasal polyposis (CRSwNP) suffer from a spectrum of disease symptoms and severities, with numerous confounding factors contributing to the disease process such as asthma, allergic rhinitis, and sleep apnea. With many variables present, a personalized approach is often needed to find the best treatment for the appropriate patient. Understanding the individual nuances of the different endotypes and characteristics of disease can allow for more precise treatment.

ENDOTYPES OF CHRONIC RHINOSINUSITIS

CRS began as a clinical syndrome that encompassed a range of disease processes that shared clinical symptoms of nasal congestion, nasal drainage, facial pain or pressure, and olfactory dysfunction.[3,4] Over the course of decades of research, identification of disease endotypes that have distinct clinical behaviors and pathophysiologies has allowed for further delineation and characterization of many forms of CRS. The first separation of disease processes within the wide umbrella of rhinosinusitis was with the identification of CRSwNP as a separate phenotypic entity from CRS without nasal polyps (CRSsNP). However, this diagnosis relies on the ability to see polyps on endoscopy or anterior rhinoscopy and may be a variable manifestation of the disease process. Polyps develop over time because of the underlying inflammatory process, often making differentiation between etiologic causes of CRSsNP and early CRSwNP impossible by physical examination alone. For example, cystic fibrosis is a genetic form of rhinosinusitis that may display a polyp phenotype but has a vastly different etiology and behavior than Th2-mediated eosinophilic CRSwNP. Endotyping of rhinosinusitis requires more information beyond appearance on nasal endoscopy or anterior rhinoscopy.

In addition to physical examination, clinical history, radiographic information, and pathophysiological data contribute to identification of subtypes of rhinosinusitis. Clinical symptoms and associated comorbidities are useful for endotyping rhinosinusitis in aspirin-exacerbated respiratory disease (AERD), which demonstrates clinical features of asthma, nasal polyps, and sensitivity to nonsteroidal anti-inflammatory drugs (NSAIDs). AERD is an endotype of CRSwNP that typically has a more recalcitrant clinical course and is amenable to treatment with aspirin desensitization.

Computed tomography (CT) scans of the sinuses are helpful in recognizing some subtypes of CRSwNP. Characteristic CT scan findings are seen in several subtypes of CRSwNP, including allergic fungal rhinosinusitis (AFRS), where there are mixed densities caused by calcifications in the fungal debris and possible bony expansion or erosion. An isolated sinus fungus ball is another type of CRS that displays CT scan findings of osteitis, opacification, and mixed densities from the fungal debris. The most recently described subtype of CRS, central compartment atopic disease (CCAD), is identified by radiographic and endoscopic features of mucosal thickening in the medial nasal structures, sparing of the peripheral sinus mucosa, and an association with inhalant allergy.[5]

Various tissue and circulating markers can be helpful in understanding endotypes of sinusitis. Inflammatory markers such as interleukin (IL)-4, IL-5, and IL-13 suggest type 2 eosinophilic inflammation.[6] The presence of purulent drainage from the sinuses with positive culture of pathogenic organisms helps identify type 1 neutrophilic inflammation. Urinary leukotrienes have been shown to aid in the diagnosis of AERD.[7] Tissue histology provides additional data with the presence of cellular populations (eosinophils vs neutrophils) or extramucosal debris (allergic mucin, fungal hyphae). Ongoing studies are attempting to determine response to medications or surgery and novel molecular markers within the sinus tissues to help subtype rhinosinusitis.

With many phenotypes of CRS and numerous clinical variables between patients, the ability to accurately diagnose, predict prognosis, and select the appropriate treatment depends on the understanding of disease subtypes and endotypes. CRS is in the early stages of disease endotyping, as a complete understanding of the disease mechanisms and endotypes within the clinical spectrum of rhinosinusitis remains unknown. With the ability of biologic medications to target specific pathways, the ability to identify endotypes is at the forefront of clinical research.

CHRONIC RHINOSINUSITIS WITH AND WITHOUT NASAL POLYPOSIS

Identification of CRSwNP compared with CRSsNP was an early distinction based on physical examination alone; however, the 2 CRS phenotypes are now differentiated by a better understanding of pathophysiological mechanisms. In Western geographic regions, CRSwNP usually manifests the eosinophilic, type 2 inflammatory mechanism by which rhinosinusitis is accompanied by polyp formation. For patients with early CRSwNP, even though frank polyps may not be seen on nasal endoscopy, the cellular findings on tissue biopsy can be consistent with CRSwNP. As mentioned previously, the presence of polyps alone does not determine the CRS subtype or endotype, as there are multiple disease processes that can display polyps. Approximately half of the patients with cystic fibrosis have nasal polyps that are formed by a much different disease process than type 2-mediated CRSwNP. Histology of cystic fibrosis polyps typically shows neutrophilic infiltrates, whereas type 2-mediated CRSwNP demonstrates eosinophilic infiltrates. Eosinophilic granulomatosis with polyangiitis (eGPA, formerly known as Churg-Strauss syndrome) is another polyp-forming disease with a distinct pathophysiologic mechanism where polyps form in the setting of eosinophilic vasculitis.

Endotyping of CRSwNP requires detailed biologic and clinical information beyond physical examination. Eosinophilia is a hallmark of type 2 inflammation, which is driven by elevation of IL-4, IL-5, and IL-13; this is distinct from the typical drivers of type 1 inflammation in CRSsNP.[6] The presence of atopic diseases, including allergic rhinitis, asthma, and atopic dermatitis, are suggestive for a systemic disease process of type 2 inflammation. Eosinophils are frequently seen in CRSwNP in the United States.[8] Circulating eosinophilia can also be a marker of CRSwNP. Eosinophil count in the blood can be calculated by taking the eosinophil percent multiplied by the total number of white blood cells.

The identification of type 2 inflammation in CRSwNP does not complete the endotyping process, as there are further classifications that differentiate disease endotypes and offer specific treatment options. As examples, AFRS, AERD, CCAD, and eosinophilic granulomatosis with polyangiitis (eGPA) demonstrate eosinophilic type 2 inflammation but have unique features with specific treatment recommendations.

AFRS is classically diagnosed by the criteria described by Bent and Kuhn,[9] which include type I immunoglobulin E (IgE)-mediated allergy to fungus, nasal polyposis, characteristic CT findings (heterogeneous intrasinus densities), allergic/eosinophilic mucin on pathology, and the presence of noninvasive fungal hyphae within the allergic mucin.[7] Surgical treatment to remove all of the fungal debris is necessary for cessation of the expansile bony changes and to help curtail the inflammatory process. Associated medical therapy includes oral and topical steroid therapy. Allergen immunotherapy may also be used as an adjunct.

AERD is an additional subtype of CRSwNP, with the addition of NSAID intolerance and asthma. AERD patients usually have a more severe and recalcitrant clinical course than NSAID-tolerant CRSwNP patients; however, the differences and similarities between disease processes are still being elucidated.[10,11] The identification of the AERD endotype allows for potential treatment with aspirin desensitization. Patients with AERD have also been shown to be particularly responsive to some biologic therapies.[11]

The most recently identified subtype of CRS is CCAD, which has a unique pattern of sinonasal inflammation in the medial regions of the sinuses, posterior nasal septum, and medial/superior turbinates and a higher association with allergic disease.[5] The lateral sparing of the sinus mucosa in early stages of CCAD is thought to be caused by medially based nasal inflammation related to allergen exposure along the usual nasal airflow patterns. Diffusely obstructed and opacified sinuses are a late finding in CCAD. The clinical impact of CCAD is not fully understood; however, counseling patients for the prognosis of persistent allergy symptoms is appropriate.

CRSsNP typically exhibits type 1 inflammation, with neutrophilic infectious or autoimmune inflammation of the sinuses. CRSsNP can be seen in conjunction with autoimmune diseases, odontogenic infections, fungus balls, immune deficiencies, ciliary dysfunction, and other idiopathic causes. The presence of purulent drainage and pain are 2 clinical characteristics that suggest CRSsNP and type 1 inflammation.[12] Less attention has been given recently to type 1 inflammation, as the treatment is aimed at the underlying cause (ie, bacterial infection, addressing dental pathology, and removal of the fungus ball) as opposed to blockade of the inflammatory cascade, with the exception of autoimmune disease such as granulomatosis with polyangiitis.

Understanding the specific pathophysiologic mechanisms of each presentation will allow for optimal treatment specific to the disease entity. As more scientific data become available regarding the pathogenesis and molecular alterations in each disease entity, there will be opportunities to correctly identify the appropriate treatments for endotypes that have overlapping clinical features.

PATIENT CHARACTERISTICS FOR SELECTING BIOLOGIC THERAPIES

Biologic therapies are currently approved for CRSwNP to block features of the type 2 inflammatory cascade. Eosinophilia is a hallmark of type 2 inflammation. As stated previously, type 2 inflammation is mediated by the cytokines IL-4, IL-5, IL-13, eosinophils, and IgE, which can be measured in blood, tissue, or secretions.[6] Although levels of serum IgE and blood eosinophils can be used to guide the use of biologic agents in the treatment of asthma,[13] there are no definitive quantitative or qualitative markers that predict the efficacy of biologics for CRSwNP.

Symptoms can be a useful marker of type 2 inflammation. Patients with a strong history of allergic diseases are likely to have type 2 inflammation associated with and/or modifying their CRSwNP. The atopic march is described as the occurrence of atopic dermatitis, food allergy, and allergic rhinitis. Approximately half of asthma patients have an allergic trigger. A history of allergic disorders may suggest that blockade of the type 2 pathway with an anti-IgE therapy like omalizumab could be beneficial for patients with CRSwNP and allergy.

There are other symptoms that have been compared between CRSwNP and CRSsNP and can aid in identification of patients who would be appropriate for treatment with type 2 blockade. The presence of purulent drainage without polyps is suggestive for type 1 inflammation. Pain and facial pressure are more suggestive of type 1 inflammation in CRSsNP.[11] The presence of olfactory dysfunction has been shown to be seen more often in CRSwNP.[14]

Biologic therapies that block type 2 inflammation are relatively new in the management of CRSwNP but have been used much longer in other atopic conditions such as asthma, chronic idiopathic urticaria, and atopic dermatitis. Although the indications for use of biologic agents in CRSwNP to date are relatively nonspecific, such as an inadequate response to nasal steroids (omalizumab) or inadequately controlled CRSwNP (dupilumab), in other atopic conditions, indications have been more specific and tailored to biomarkers or patient characteristics. The European Forum for Research and Education in Allergy and Airway Diseases (EUFOREA) has proposed criteria for biologic therapy suggesting that patients have undergone prior endoscopic sinus surgery (ESS) and meet 3 of the following 5 criteria: type 2 inflammatory profile, need for systemic steroids in the past 2 years, significant quality of life impairment, significant smell loss, and diagnosis of comorbid asthma. Additionally, they have recommended evaluation of treatment at 16 weeks and 1 year in order to limit expense and exposure in nonresponding patients.[15]

Dupilumab is indicated for glucocorticoid-dependent asthma or eosinophilic asthma as it has shown particular efficacy in these groups.[16,17] In those studies, patients were required to be on chronic oral glucocorticosteroids or to have serum eosinophil count of at least 300 cells per microliter and sputum eosinophilia of at least 3%, and patients with these characteristics did well on dupilumab, decreasing dependence on glucocorticosteroids and improving lung function parameters.[16,17] Similarly, in asthma, omalizumab has been shown to be effective for patients with elevation in total IgE and specific perennial allergen sensitization whose symptoms are uncontrolled on inhaled corticosteroids.

When determining clinical features that would suggest appropriate treatment with biologic therapies, information can also be obtained from the inclusion and exclusion criteria in clinical trials. A large randomized controlled trial of dupilumab for CRSwNP included patients older than 18 years with bilateral disease, a high polyp burden, and a more severe phenotype.[1] Half of the subjects had asthma or AERD. Excluded from study were subjects who had antrochoanal nasal polyps, acute rhinosinusitis, upper respiratory infection, allergic granulomatous angiitis/eosinophilic granulomatosis with polyangiitis, granulomatosis with polyangiitis, cystic fibrosis, fungal rhinosinusitis, Young syndrome, Kartagener syndrome, or dyskinetic cilia syndrome.[1]

For a large randomized controlled trial of omalizumab, adult patients with bilateral, severe diseases with serum IgE between 30 and 1500 IU/mL were eligible.[2] Patients were excluded if they had current upper respiratory tract infection; cystic fibrosis; dyskinetic ciliary syndrome; malignancy; cardiac condition; hepatitis; liver cirrhosis; recent or current infection requiring hospitalization; antibiotic or antifungal treatment; parasitic infection; use of systemic corticosteroids within the past 2 months; use of immunosuppressant, biologic, or leukotriene antagonist or modifier; recent nasal surgery, or immunocompromised state.[2]

As discussed previously, like asthma, CRSwNP is a heterogenous disease with multiple subtypes and endotypes that present in similar fashion or phenotype. Specific biomarkers will need to be identified to help stratify patients beyond current understanding. This will guide future decision making for whether patients should initiate biologic therapy (and which biologic agent), continue medical management, or pursue ESS.

DEFINING FAILURES OF STANDARD THERAPY

CRSwNP is known to have a significant impact on quality of life, with patients with chronic rhinosinusitis having health utility values lower than many other significant diseases including congestive heart failure and chronic obstructive pulmonary disease.[18,19] It has been demonstrated through prospective study that some patients will improve through initial medical treatment with topical nasal steroids and sinus irrigations, but a high percentage will have significant disease burden even after initial medical therapy.[20] The concept of maximal medical therapy for chronic rhinosinusitis has shifted to a concept of appropriate medical therapy, acknowledging that the number of medical therapies has increased dramatically.[21]

For patients who do not improve with medical therapy, ESS has been demonstrated to have significant improvement in quality of life and is likely superior to continued medical management.[22] ESS has been shown to improve health utility value from significant impairment to those that approximate the general US population with durable results over many years, suggesting that ESS is a viable option for medically refractory patients.[18] Primary and revision sinus surgery have demonstrated significant improvement from baseline in the long term, again suggesting that surgery is reasonable for patients with significant impairment even if they have had surgery in the past.[18]

Standard therapy for CRSwNP is generally well described.[3,4] Defining failure of standard therapy and consideration for use of biologic therapies is not well characterized in the literature or in US Food and Drug Administration (FDA) labeling of biologic therapies. Insight can be obtained from a traditional teaching regarding failure of appropriate medical therapies as an indication for sinus surgery. There are a range of acceptable medical therapies, and individual patient characteristics and preferences often determine when it is appropriate for a patient to elect sinus surgery. Although the relationship between use of biologic agents and sinus surgery will likely remain controversial until more studies are presented, the subjective nature of the clinical severity of patient symptoms will likely limit strict guidelines in the future.

In trials of dupilumab, it has been shown that there is significant reduction of nasal polyp scores and symptoms of nasal obstruction. However, if the monoclonal antibody is stopped, polyps recur and symptoms worsen toward baseline.[1] Given the success of ESS in many refractory patients and the need for seemingly long-term monoclonal antibody treatment, ESS should first be considered in patients who fail appropriate medical therapy. As suggested by the EUFOREA criteria, biologic treatment can be considered for patients who have refractory disease despite comprehensive surgery.[15] It may also be considered in patients who are poor surgical candidates, or have comorbid conditions that may benefit from a biologic agent known to improve CRSwNP.

Additionally, cost analysis has demonstrated that, when comparing ESS to treatment with dupilumab for CRSwNP, sinus surgery produces more quality-adjusted life years (QALYs) and is less expensive than dupilumab, although both produced QALYs. Given that surgery is effective in medically refractory patients (including those who are undergoing revision surgery), produces more QALYs, and is less expensive than current biologic therapy, surgery remains an appealing option before committing to a long-term medication with high cost.[23]

Patient-centered decision making is an important principle in determining the appropriate decision for a patient undergoing biologic therapy versus sinus surgery. Having an informed consent process is essential to utilizing patient-centered decision making. Helping patients to understand that a large percentage will be able to avoid life-long biologic medications with ESS, and that medical therapy is available for refractory cases that meet criteria such as those laid out by the EUFOREA group is important to guiding patients through care of this chronic condition. For patients who are not acceptable candidates for general anesthesia, biologic therapies may also be a viable option as was demonstrated in the clinical trials.

SUMMARY

Endotyping/subtyping of CRSwNP uses clinical information, radiographic studies, and pathophysiologic data to understand the pathologic mechanism driving the inflammatory cascade. Understanding the full spectrum of chronic rhinosinusitis is in its infancy, but recent identification of disease endotypes in conjunction with the availability of biologic therapies to inhibit specific pathways provides much hope for improvements in CRSwNP treatments. A personalized approach to treatment will consider standard medical therapies, sinus surgeries, and targeted use of biologics for informed patients with the appropriate endotype/subtype characteristics.

CLINICS CARE POINTS

- Rhinosinusitis work-up should include identification of features suggestive for specific endotypes and subtypes. Biologic and clinical information, physical examination, radiographic studies, tissue histology, and other adjunct markers of inflammation should be sought to understand variations in disease type that can impact treatment options.
- The severity of disease and response to treatment for patients with rhinosinusitis should be monitored to determine which patients would benefit from additional treatment options. Biologic treatment for patients with nasal polyps should be considered for patients who have refractory disease despite appropriate medical therapy, and comprehensive surgery, or who are poor surgical candidates or have comorbid conditions such as asthma.

DISCLOSURE

M.P. Platt and C.D. Brook are consultants for GI Reviewers, LLC.

REFERENCES

1. Bachert C, Han JK, Desrosiers M, et al. Efficacy and safety of dupilumab in patients with severe chronic rhinosinusitis with nasal polyps (LIBERTY NP SINUS-24 and LIBERTY NP SINUS-52): results from two multicentre, randomised, double-blind, placebo-controlled, parallel-group phase 3 trials. Lancet 2019;394:1638–50.
2. Gevaert P, Omachi TA, Corren J, et al. Efficacy and safety of omalizumab in nasal polyposis: 2 randomized phase 3 trials. J Allergy Clin Immunol 2020;146(3):595–605. Erratum in: J Allergy Clin Immunol. 2021 Jan;147(1):416. PMID: 32524991.
3. Orlandi RR, Kingdom TT, Hwang PH, et al. International consensus statement on allergy and rhinology: rhinosinusitis. Int Forum Allergy Rhinol 2016;6(Suppl 1):S22–209.
4. Fokkens WJ, Lund VJ, Hopkins C, et al. European position paper on rhinosinusitis and Nasal Polyps 2020. Rhinology 2020;58(Suppl S29):1–464.
5. DelGaudio JM, Loftus PA, Hamizan AW, et al. Central compartment atopic disease. Am J Rhinol Allergy 2017;31(4):228–34.
6. Damask CC, Ryan MW, Casale TB, et al. Targeted molecular therapies in allergy and rhinology. Otolaryngol Head Neck Surg 2021;164(Suppl 1):S1–21.
7. Bochenek G, Stachura T, Szafraniec K, et al. Diagnostic accuracy of urinary lte4 measurement to predict aspirin-exacerbated respiratory disease in patients with asthma. J Allergy Clin Immunol Pract 2018;6(2):528–35.

8. Pan L, Liao B, Guo CL, et al. Inflammatory features and predictors for postsurgical outcomes in patients with nasal polyps stratified by local and systemic eosinophilia. Int Forum Allergy Rhinol 2020. https://doi.org/10.1002/alr.22702.
9. Bent JP 3rd, Kuhn FA. Diagnosis of allergic fungal sinusitis. Otolaryngol Head Neck Surg 1994;111(5):580–8.
10. Mustafa SS, Vadamalai K, Scott B, et al. Dupilumab as add-on therapy for chronic rhinosinusitis with nasal polyposis in aspirin exacerbated respiratory disease. Am J Rhinol Allergy 2020;35(3):399–407.
11. Laidlaw TM, Mullol J, Fan C, et al. Dupilumab improves nasal polyp burden and asthma control in patients with CRSwNP and AERD. J Allergy Clin Immunol Pract 2019;7(7):2462–5.e1.
12. Jones NS. The prevalence of facial pain and purulent sinusitis. Curr Opin Otolaryngol Head Neck Surg 2009;17(1):38–42.
13. Castro M, Corren J, Pavord ID, et al. Dupilumab efficacy and safety in moderate-to-severe uncontrolled asthma. N Engl J Med 2018;378:2486–96.
14. Stevens WW, Peters AT, Tan BK, et al. Associations between inflammatory endotypes and clinical presentations in chronic rhinosinusitis. J Allergy Clin Immunol Pract 2019;7(8):2812–20.e3.
15. Fokkens WJ, Lund V, Bachert C, et al. EUFOREA consensus on biologics for CRSwNP with or without asthma. Allergy 2019;74(12):2312–9.
16. Rabe KF, Nair P, Brusselle G, et al. Efficacy and safety of dupilumab in glucocorticoid-dependent severe asthma. N Engl J Med 2018;378(26):2475–85.
17. Wenzel S, Ford L, Pearlman D, et al. Dupilumab in persistent asthma with elevated eosinophil levels. N Engl J Med 2013;368(26):2455–66.
18. Rudmik L, Mace J, Soler ZM, et al. Long-term utility outcomes in patients undergoing endoscopic sinus surgery. Laryngoscope 2014;124(1):19–23.
19. Soler ZM, Wittenberg E, Schlosser RJ, et al. Health state utility values in patients undergoing endoscopic sinus surgery. Laryngoscope 2011;121:2672–8.
20. Ragab SM, Lund VJ, Scadding G. Evaluation of the medical and surgical treatment of chronic rhinosinusitis: a prospective, randomised, controlled trial. Laryngoscope 2004;114(5):923–30.
21. Rudmik L, Soler ZM, Hopkins C, et al. Defining appropriateness criteria for endoscopic sinus surgery during management of uncomplicated adult chronic rhinosinusitis: a RAND/UCLA appropriateness study. Int Forum Allergy Rhinol 2016;6(6):557–67.
22. Patel ZM, Thamboo A, Rudmik L, et al. Surgical therapy vs continued medical therapy for medically refractory chronic rhinosinusitis: a systematic review and meta-analysis. Int Forum Allergy Rhinol 2017;7(2):119–27.
23. Scangas GA, Wu AW, Ting JY, et al. Cost utility analysis of dupilumab versus endoscopic sinus surgery for chronic rhinosinusitis with nasal polyps. Laryngoscope 2020. https://doi.org/10.1002/lary.28648.

Knowledge Gaps and Research Needs for Biologic Therapy in Rhinology Practice

Lauren T. Roland, MD, MSCI[a], Joshua M. Levy, MD, MPH[b,*]

KEYWORDS

- Biologic agents • Chronic rhinosinusitis with nasal polyps
- Aspirin-exacerbated respiratory disease

KEY POINTS

- Indications for use of biologic agents in various chronic rhinosinusitis with nasal polyposis (CRSwNP) endotypes need to be clearly defined.
- Biomarkers associated with a clinically meaningful response to biologic therapies are needed to facilitate appropriate patient selection.
- Head-to-head trials will be needed to compare outcomes of various biologic agents for CRSwNP.
- Required duration of biologic therapy needs to be assessed.
- Cost-effectiveness analyses are needed to determine an appropriate treatment algorithm.

INTRODUCTION/HISTORY/DEFINITIONS/BACKGROUND

Chronic rhinosinusitis (CRS) is a form of sinonasal inflammation with unmet needs for patient treatment, especially in those with recalcitrant disease. The prevalence of CRS is between 5% and 16%,[1] with nasal polyps (CRSwNP) occurring in about 25% of cases.[2] The economic burden of CRS treatment is estimated to be approximately $22 billion per year in the United States.[1] CRS patients are a heterogeneous group represented by several inflammatory endotypes. Among these, the most common CRSwNP endotypes are defined by high levels of type-2 inflammatory mediators, including eosinophilic CRSwNP, aspirin-exacerbated respiratory disease (AERD), allergic fungal rhinosinusitis (AFRS), and central compartment atopic disease (CCAD).[3,4] Current treatment options for all CRS endotypes include appropriate medical management with topical saline irrigations and intranasal corticosteroids, as well

[a] Otolaryngology–Head and Neck Surgery, University of California, San Francisco, 2233 Post Street, Box 1225, San Francisco, CA 94115, USA; [b] Otolaryngology–Head and Neck Surgery, Emory Sinus, Nasal and Allergy Center, 550 Peachtree Street NE, MOT Building, Suite 1135, Atlanta, GA 30308, USA
* Corresponding author.
E-mail address: joshua.levy2@emory.edu

Otolaryngol Clin N Am 54 (2021) 709–716
https://doi.org/10.1016/j.otc.2021.04.002
0030-6665/21/

as oral corticosteroids or antibiotics as medically indicated. Endoscopic sinus surgery (ESS) is subsequently considered to remove obstructive tissue and facilitate the postoperative delivery of topical medications. However, despite adherence to contemporary treatment guidelines, the rates of disease recurrence following ESS remains high.[5] Innovative treatment strategies are therefore needed to improve patient care for this recalcitrant disease.

Biologic agents are humanized monoclonal antibodies designed to act upon a specific target, such as specific Th-2 mediators/receptors (eg, immunoglobulin E [IgE], interleukin [IL]-5 and IL-5Rα, IL-4Rα) associated with many forms of CRSwNP.[6] By targeting specific pathways of the inflammatory response, biologic medications have shown promising results for multiple diseases including asthma, atopic dermatitis and CRSwNP.[7] In June 2019, dupilumab was the first biologic approved for use in CRSwNP patients, and omalizumab was approved for use in CRSwNP in December 2020. There are several other biologics currently under investigation for potential approval for the CRSwNP indication in the near future.

NATURE OF THE PROBLEM

Despite studies suggesting multiple objective and patient-reported benefits of biologic agents as an adjunctive treatment for CRSwNP, several unanswered questions remain. These questions are challenging to investigate because of the immunologic complexity and heterogeneity of CRSwNP patients. Additionally, when attempting to compare biologic agents with other management options, blinding patients and physicians becomes nearly impossible, particularly because surgery is a potential treatment for recalcitrant CRSwNP. Nonetheless, research investigating the current gaps in knowledge for biologic agents in a rhinology practice is critical. Overall, the most important research need is to determine the best treatment algorithm for each unique patient. Treatment algorithms should be determined by patient outcomes and cost-effectiveness analyses.

Patients have options regarding their care for CRSwNP and should consider the risks, benefits, and alternatives to all treatment options. At this point, quality-of-life outcomes have not been well studied for comparison of biologic agents with other CRSwNP treatment regimens, such as aspirin desensitization and high-dose maintenance aspirin therapy for AERD. Additionally, the efficacy of various treatment algorithms, including the timing of surgical intervention and biologic agent administration, has not been compared. By furthering these areas of investigation, counseling patients on treatment choices would become supported by evidence-based medicine.

Biologic agents, which are currently costly, are likely to be long-term or even lifelong medications. Prior work has suggested that surgery is cost-effective when compared with biologic agents for the initial treatment of CRSwNP.[8] However, cost-effectiveness studies are lacking to evaluate the economic effects of incorporating biologic agents as an option after a patient has failed a primary surgery. Additionally, the heterogeneous group of CRSwNP patients should be assessed to determine which patients, if any, have long-lasting efficacy if biologic agents are stopped. More work is needed to characterize biomarkers to identify patients who will best respond to biologics, making biologic agents a potentially more cost-effective option compared with multiple surgeries and other medical management.[9]

In November 2019, the National Institutes of Health (NIH) hosted a meeting to promote discussion among experts in industry and the fields of rhinology, pulmonary medicine, allergy/immunology, and statistics. This discussion identified several critical research needs for the study of biologic agents in CRSwNP patients.[10] The group acknowledged that the primary goal of studies moving forward is to determine where biologic agents belong within the treatment algorithm. Several topics of discussion were raised, including how to measure success (through patient-reported outcomes, imaging, endoscopy findings, or biomarkers) and the challenges of inclusion and exclusion criteria when studying a heterogeneous group of patients, while still maintaining generalizability of data.[10]

CURRENT EVIDENCE

The current evidence supporting biologic agents in CRSwNP is discussed in more detail in Ramaswamy and colleagues' article, "Current Evidence for Biologic Therapy in Chronic Rhinosinusitis with Nasal Polyposis," by in this issue. Briefly, dupilumab, which targets the effects of IL-4 and IL-13 by targeting the IL-4 α-receptor shared by these 2 cytokines, was approved for use in CRSwNP patients in 2019. Dupilumab has been shown to improve polyp scores and quality-of-life measures.[11] Omalizumab, an anti-IgE agent, was approved for use in polyp patients in December 2020. Studies suggest improvement of clinical, endoscopic, and quality-of-life measures.[12] There are several other biologic agents approved for use in other Th2-mediated respiratory diseases, such as asthma, as well as newer biologic agents under investigation. Likely, biologic agents with other targets, such IL-5 and its receptor, will become available for the CRSwNP indication.[7]

GUIDANCE FOR TREATMENT

Several documents contain initial guidance for otolaryngologists regarding the use of biologics in CRSwNP. A group of rhinologists and allergists from the United States recently proposed a treatment algorithm for CRSwNP patients after the research-focused NIH discussion revealed little evidence-based guidance for current treatment planning.[13] These experts advocated consideration of biologic agents as a treatment option after a patient fails both medical management and ESS with postoperative oral and topical corticosteroids. The document also stressed the importance of evaluating patients at 4 months for improvement on these medications. This timeline is similar to the evaluation period suggested for biologic agents in asthma patients.[14] Evaluation for initial benefit of biologic therapy in CRSwNP may include nasal endoscopy, investigation of sinonasal quality-of-life measures, and the need for medications for sinus and respiratory symptoms.[13]

European guidance states that biologic agents should be considered for patients who have had surgery and meet any 3 of the following criteria: type 2 inflammation, 2 or more courses of oral steroids within 1 year, impaired quality of life, loss of smell, and comorbid asthma. For patients who have not undergone surgery, 4 or more of the criteria must be met before considering biologic agents for CRSwNP.[15] As more data become available, recommendations for specific patient populations will likely change.

CONTROVERSIES

Controversies regarding the care of CRSwNP patients are primarily focused on delineating the most appropriate treatment algorithm. In present times, proposed treatment algorithms are largely based on expert opinion, and will evolve with emerging evidence and as more biologic agents become US Food and Drug Administration

(FDA) approved for the CRSwNP indication. One area of dispute is if biologic agents should be prescribed to patients before consideration of surgery. Although some advocate for considering biologic agents only after a surgical intervention, there may be some situations in which surgery or anesthesia is not feasible or appropriate. Future evaluation of biologic agents as a postoperative adjuvant therapy for patients with persistent sinonasal inflammation after ESS will add critical information in this regard. Although the concept of a medical polypectomy or use of a biologic agent to comprehensively remove established polyp tissue is not supported by current phase 3 trials, the efficacy of these medications in reversing the early recurrence of disease remains a concept with the potential to greatly decrease the need for revision ESS.

Another area of controversy to consider is the appropriate prescriber for each indication of biologic agents. As biologic agents have been approved and used for treatment of asthma and other Th-2 mediated processes for several years, allergy, immunology, and pulmonary physicians have extensive experience prescribing these medications. Many CRSwNP patients have a comorbid asthma diagnosis and will be followed by both an otolaryngologist and a medical specialist. As indications for biologic agents expand, there will be a need to closely work together to communicate regarding these complicated patients. Each specialist has expertise in unique diagnostic tools (eg, nasal endoscopy and pulmonary function testing), and while controversies regarding appropriate patient selection for biologic agents may arise, there will be significant benefit from collaboration.

The current Coronavirus disease 2019 (COVID-19) pandemic has also led to questions regarding the safety of biologic agents during these unexpected times. A rare adverse effect of Th2-associated biologic agents is a helminthic infection, and there is a technical possibility of an increased susceptibility to COVID-19 or other respiratory viral pathogens while taking these immune-modulating medications.[16] A recent study has shown a decrease in ACE2 receptors, the site of severe acute respiratory syndrome coronavirus 2 (SARS-CoV-2) host entry, in polyp tissue compared with sinonasal tissue from patients without CRSwNP.[17] Another recent study suggested that patients on multiple biologics for psoriasis management did show an increased risk of COVID infection but had decreased risk of severe COVID symptoms, potentially because of the effects of biologic agents acting to block a cytokine storm.[18] Compared with surgery, some biologic agents can be administered at home, avoiding contact with others, which may be beneficial during this time. As with most research areas regarding the current pandemic, there is still much to learn about the relationship between biologic agents and COVID-19. Additional work to understand the potential effects of immune modulators on host response to vaccination will also be needed.

DISCUSSION

This section discusses several research needs for biologic therapy in rhinology practice in order to develop evidence-based treatment algorithm recommendations (**Table 1**).

Biomarkers: Identifying the Right Drug, for the Right Patient, at the Right Time

Biomarkers are measurable clinical factors that may aid in disease diagnosis or the prediction of a therapeutic response. Biomarkers are critical to predict the success of biologic therapies in an individual patient with CRS. Uniform and objective measures across studies are needed and may be measurable from any biologic source. Although several biomarkers for the identification of specific CRSwNP endotypes,

Table 1
Research needs

Area of Research	Specific Questions
Biomarkers	• Which biomarkers should be used to define eligibility for biologic agents? • How can success of biologic treatment be measured using biomarkers? • Can biomarkers be used to determine if patients can wean or stop biologic therapy?
Endotype/phenotype	• How do biologic agents perform in nested analyses of CRSwNP subgroups?
Clinical trials – head-to-head comparisons	• How do biologic agents compare to one another in terms of symptom improvement, tolerance, and safety?
CRSsNP	• Are biologic agents efficacious in patients without nasal polyps? • Is biologic efficacy dependent on allergy/atopic state?
Cost-effectiveness	• For which patients are biologics considered cost-effective? • At what point does biologic therapy become cost-effective compared with revision surgery?
AERD	• How does aspirin desensitization compare with biologic agents in AERD patients? • Which treatment option is better tolerated by patients – biologic therapy or maintenance aspirin therapy? • Is there any benefit to combining aspirin therapy with biologic agents for the most recalcitrant patients?

such as AERD, have been described, a predictive biomarker for response to biologic therapies has yet to be described.[19,20] This is a critical need to identify patients with the greatest likelihood of experiencing a clinically important treatment response.

Endotype/Phenotype

It is accepted that there are several unique endotypes and phenotypes of CRS.[21] Likely, specific molecular antibody targets are most appropriate for distinct subtypes of CRS. Biomarkers, as discussed previously, will be useful for a deeper understanding of subtypes of disease. Further work investigating the true delineation of CRS patients, beyond CRSwNP and CRSsNP, will also advance the understanding of appropriate biologic therapy for each individual patient.[21] Studies should include all CRSwNP patients, but also be powered for separate analyses of subgroups of patients to understand indications for specific patients. For example, the nested analysis of the dupilumab phase 2a clinical trial (NCT01920893) showed several superior outcomes among subjects with AERD versus those without aspirin sensitivity.[22] Additionally, some nasal polyp endotypes, such as AFRS, have been largely excluded from prior clinical study and require further investigation.[11]

Head-to-Head Trials

Once more biologic options exist for CRSwNP patients, there will be a need to compare options in head-to-head blinded trials. These trials will allow for a direct comparison of biologics options with similar but slightly variable targets within the inflammatory pathway. This work may also allow the identification of patient or polyp characteristics, which respond in a more significant way to a specific biologic agent.

Most work has focused on CRSwNP patients, and biologic agents have not been well studied in patients with CRSsNP.[23] The benefit of biologic agents in these patients is unknown, and the association with allergy and Th-2 mediated disease is less clear.[24]

Cost-Effectiveness

Cost-effectiveness analyses should include direct costs of surgery and medications and indirect costs such as missed work caused by illness or treatment requirements. Quality-of-life measurements and patient preference will also contribute greatly to these analyses.

Treatment Options - Biologic Agents Versus Aspirin Desensitization

Several studies have suggested the benefit of aspirin desensitization in AERD patients regarding subjective quality-of-life improvement and a decrease in polyp burden and need for revision surgery.[25] Maintenance aspirin therapy is a lifelong treatment, and while inexpensive, it is associated with adverse effects.[26] A comparison of aspirin therapy and biologic agents in regards to efficacy and quality-of-life outcomes in AERD patients is warranted. This work will be especially interesting, as these management strategies are both long-term treatment options, but vary greatly in direct costs.

FUTURE DIRECTIONS

There are several ongoing trials to assess various biologics in CRSwNP patients. These studies are assessing both CRSwNP patients in general, and specific subsets of CRSwNP. Given that there is still much to learn regarding endotypes and phenotypes of CRSwNP and biomarkers to predict a clinical response, this area of research will be ongoing for many years. It is particularly challenging to determine the external validity of CRS studies, as CRSwNP patients are known to be heterogeneous regarding biomarkers, allergic status, polyp size, computed tomography findings, and subjective quality of life. On a larger scale, it would be beneficial to consider a multi-institutional registry of CRSwNP patients to include investigation of outcomes and polyp tissue from participants around the world.[10] Ultimately, work in this field will lead to more complete and evidence-based treatment recommendations to guide physicians caring for these complicated patients.

SUMMARY

Biologic agents are an emerging therapeutic option for patients with recalcitrant sinus disease. Although pivotal phase 3 trials consistently demonstrate clinically important differences in several objective and patient reported outcomes following biologic treatment for CRSwNP, additional investigations are needed to define their appropriate use. Future study aimed at discovering predictive biomarkers will greatly aid in patient identification, while evaluation of efficacy in the postoperative setting will further define treatment indications. Finally, evaluation of specific CRSwNP endotypes, such as AFRS, will fill existing gaps in the literature and provide evidence for a greater number of patients with persistent sinonasal disease.

CLINICS CARE POINTS

- Biologic agents have recently become approved for use in CRSwNP patients.
- Biologic agent use in specific CRSwNP endotypes needs to be studied to determine appropriate patient selection.

- Uniform use of biomarkers and clinical outcome measures should be incorporated to study clinical improvement.
- Cost-effectiveness studies are currently a critical unmet need.

DISCLOSURE

L.T. Roland – Tissium (consultant), NeurENT (research support); J.M. Levy - Clinical Research: AstraZeneca, Cumberland Pharmaceuticals, Gossammer Bio, Inc., Sanofi/Regeneron and OptiNose. Advisory board: AstraZeneca and Sanofi/Regeneron.

REFERENCES

1. Smith KA, Orlandi RR, Rudmik L. Cost of adult chronic rhinosinusitis: a systematic review. Laryngoscope 2015;125(7):1547–56.
2. Stevens WW, Schleimer RP, Kern RC. Chronic rhinosinusitis with nasal polyps. J Allergy Clin Immunol Pract 2016;4(4):565–72.
3. Koennecke M, Klimek L, Mullol J, et al. Subtyping of polyposis nasi: phenotypes, endotypes and comorbidities. Allergo J Int 2018;27(2):56–65.
4. DelGaudio JM, Loftus PA, Hamizan AW, et al. Central compartment atopic disease. Am J Rhinol Allergy 2017;31(4):228–34.
5. DeConde AS, Mace JC, Levy JM, et al. Prevalence of polyp recurrence after endoscopic sinus surgery for chronic rhinosinusitis with nasal polyposis. Laryngoscope 2017;127(3):550–5.
6. Damask CC, Ryan MW, Casale TB, et al. Targeted molecular therapies in allergy and rhinology. Otolaryngol Head Neck Surg 2020;164(suppl 1):S1–21.
7. Kim C, Han J, Wu T, et al. Role of biologics in chronic rhinosinusitis with nasal polyposis: state of the art review. Otolaryngol Head Neck Surg 2020;164(1):57–66.
8. Scangas GA, Wu AW, Ting JY, et al. Cost utility analysis of dupilumab versus endoscopic sinus surgery for chronic rhinosinusitis with nasal polyps. Laryngoscope 2020;131(1):E26–E33..
9. Codispoti CD, Mahdavinia M. A call for cost-effectiveness analysis for biologic therapies in chronic rhinosinusitis with nasal polyps. Ann Allergy Asthma Immunol 2019;123(3):232–9.
10. Naclerio R, Baroody F, Bachert C, et al. Clinical research needs for the management of chronic rhinosinusitis with nasal polyps in the new era of biologics. a national institute of allergy and infectious diseases workshop. J Allergy Clin Immunol Pract 2020;8(5):1532–49.e1.
11. Bachert C, et al. Efficacy and safety of dupilumab in patients with severe chronic rhinosinusitis with nasal polyps (LIBERTY NP SINUS-24 and LIBERTY NP SINUS-52): results from two multicentre, randomised, double-blind, placebo-controlled, parallel-group phase 3 trials. Lancet 2019;394:1638–1650..
12. Gevaert P, Omachi TA, Corren J, et al. Efficacy and safety of omalizumab in nasal polyposis: 2 randomized phase 3 trials. J Allergy Clin Immunol 2020;146(3):595–605.
13. Roland LT, Smith TL, Schlosser RJ, et al. Guidance for contemporary use of biologics in management of chronic rhinosinusitis with nasal polyps: discussion from a National Institutes of Health-sponsored workshop. Int Forum Allergy Rhinol 2020;10(9):1037–42.

14. Bousquet J, Brusselle G, Buhl R, et al. Care pathways for the selection of a biologic in severe asthma. Eur Respir J 2017;50(6):1701782.
15. Fokkens WJ, Lund V, Bachert C, et al. EUFOREA consensus on biologics for CRSwNP with or without asthma. Allergy 2019;74(12):2312–9.
16. Roland LT, Pinto JM, Naclerio RM. The treatment paradigm of chronic rhinosinusitis with nasal polyps in the COVD-19 Era. J Allergy Clin Immunol Pract 2020; 8(8):2492–4.
17. Jian L, Yi W, Zhang N, et al. Perspective: COVID-19, implications of nasal diseases and consequences for their management. J Allergy Clin Immunol 2020; 146(1):67–9.
18. Damiani G, Pacifico A, Bragazzi NL, et al. Biologics increase the risk of SARS-CoV-2 infection and hospitalization, but not ICU admission and death: Real-life data from a large cohort during red-zone declaration. Dermatol Ther 2020;33: e13475.
19. Corrado A, Battle M, Wise SK, et al. Endocannabinoid receptor CB2R is significantly expressed in aspirin-exacerbated respiratory disease: a pilot study. Int Forum Allergy Rhinol 2018;8(10):1184–9.
20. Choby G, O'Brien EK, Smith A, et al. Elevated Urine Leukotriene E4 is associated with worse objective markers in nasal polyposis patients. Laryngoscope 2020; 131(5):961–6.
21. Grayson JW, Hopkins C, Mori E, et al. Contemporary classification of chronic rhinosinusitis beyond polyps vs no polyps: a review. JAMA Otolaryngol Head Neck Surg 2020;146(9):831–8.
22. Laidlaw TM, Mullol J, Fan C, et al. Dupilumab improves nasal polyp burden and asthma control in patients with CRSwNP and AERD. J Allergy Clin Immunol Pract 2019;7(7):2462–5.e1.
23. Iqbal IZ, Kao SS, Ooi EH. The role of biologics in chronic rhinosinusitis: a systematic review. Int Forum Allergy Rhinol 2020;10(2):165–74.
24. Marcus S, Roland LT, DelGaudio JM, et al. The relationship between allergy and chronic rhinosinusitis. Laryngoscope Investig Otolaryngol 2019;4(1):13–7.
25. Adappa ND, Ranasinghe VJ, Trope M, et al. Outcomes after complete endoscopic sinus surgery and aspirin desensitization in aspirin-exacerbated respiratory disease. Int Forum Allergy Rhinol 2018;8(1):49–53.
26. Berges-Gimeno MP, Simon RA, Stevenson DD. Long-term treatment with aspirin desensitization in asthmatic patients with aspirin-exacerbated respiratory disease. J Allergy Clin Immunol 2003;111(1):180–6.

Mechanisms and Practical Use of Biologic Therapies for Allergy and Asthma Indications

Cecelia Damask, DO[a], Christine Franzese, MD[b,*]

KEYWORDS

• Biologic agent • Allergic rhinitis • Asthma • Anti-IgE • Anti–IL-5 • Anti–IL-4 • Anti–IL-13 • Anti-TSLP

KEY POINTS

- Currently available biologics for allergy and asthma are monoclonal antibodies that target specific cytokines or receptors in the type 2 inflammatory cascade.
- These agents have the potential to treat more than 1 disease process because of shared inflammatory pathways and downstream effects.
- Understanding the pathophysiology behind asthma and atopic disorders can help with patient selection for these agents.
- Practicalities, such as frequency of injection, disease endotype/phenotype, weight-based dosing, and other considerations, are also important when considering the use of monoclonal antibodies for allergy and asthma indications.

INTRODUCTION

Over the last 2 decades, the understanding of the immune mechanisms in inflammatory disorders has increased and the different atopic and nonatopic pathways that contribute to various endotypes of asthma and other allergic diseases have been further elucidated. Since the first biologic agent for asthma gained approval from the US Food and Drug Administration (FDA), interest in the development of additional agents to other potential immunologic targets has increased; with this peaked attention, further monoclonal antibodies have received FDA approval for asthma and other diseases. Because these novel therapeutics target different cytokines and cytokine receptors at different points in the inflammatory cascade, they have the potential to treat several different, and perhaps seemingly unrelated, disorders. The potential to treat more than 1 disorder with the same agent is appealing, but these therapies have

[a] Lake Mary Ear, Nose, Throat, and Allergy, 795 Primera Boulevard, Suite 1031, Lake Mary, FL 32746, USA; [b] Department of Otolaryngology-Head and Neck Surgery, University of Missouri-Columbia, One Hospital Drive, Suite MA314, Columbia, MO 65212, USA
* Corresponding author.
E-mail address: franzesec@health.missouri.edu

Otolaryngol Clin N Am 54 (2021) 717–728
https://doi.org/10.1016/j.otc.2021.04.003 oto.theclinics.com

significant costs or potential side effects. Understanding inflammatory biomarkers, patient profiles, and immunologic targets can assist physicians with patient and agent selection. This article presents a discussion of the current and some future biologic agents available for use in treating allergies and asthma.

DISCUSSION

Allergy is an immense subject, spanning diseases from food allergy to allergic contact dermatitis, and involving different types of hypersensitivity reactions. A discussion of all the available biologic agents for the scope of allergy is beyond this single article, and some of these disorders are addressed elsewhere in this issue. In this article, the subject of allergy is limited to addressing allergic rhinitis caused by type I immunoglobulin (Ig) E–mediated hypersensitivity, and does not include allergy caused by foods, medications, or other agents.

Allergic rhinitis is mediated by specific IgE directed against allergens. This process involves expression of cytokines, specifically interleukin (IL)-4, IL-5, and IL-13, associated with T-helper 2 (Th2) effector cells as well as infiltration of eosinophils, basophils, mast cells, and other inflammatory cells present in this type 2 inflammatory disease. Different types of inflammation are recognized and at least 3 different types of inflammation (type 1, type 2, and type 3) have been described, with type 2 immune mechanisms underlying most allergic disorders.[1–3] The presence of these type 2 cytokines in allergic rhinitis has led to the investigation of using biologics developed for other type 2 diseases, such as asthma and chronic rhinosinusitis with nasal polyposis, as treatment options in allergic rhinitis.

BIOLOGICS FOR ALLERGY

At present, there are no FDA-approved biologic options for the treatment of allergic rhinitis; however, there are biologics currently in the development pipeline, in phase III trials, or available for other FDA-approved indications that have been studied for the treatment of allergic rhinitis to environmental inhalants. In addition to current agents targeting cytokines, monoclonal antibodies targeting specific epitopes on certain allergens, such as cat or birch, are presently under investigation. However, because no specific agent is currently available for the treatment of allergic rhinitis alone, the practical applications of available therapeutics are limited and require the presence of a comorbidity that meets an FDA-approved biologic indication.

Omalizumab

Cross-linking of surface IgE and the resulting mast cell and basophil degranulation lead to the release of vasoactive and other proinflammatory mediators that result in the symptoms associated with allergic rhinitis, namely rhinorrhea, pruritus, sneezing, and so forth. The mechanism of action for omalizumab (tradename: Xolair) is further discussed later in the article, but, in summary, it is a humanized monoclonal anti-IgE antibody that binds to serum IgE molecules and has the subsequent downstream effect of reducing surface IgE cross-linking. Currently FDA approved for other indications, omalizumab has been studied for the treatment of allergic rhinitis both as a direct and as an add-on therapy.

A recent meta-analysis assessed the efficacy and safety of omalizumab in the treatment of allergic rhinitis.[4] Sixteen randomized controlled studies on the treatment of allergic rhinitis with omalizumab were identified by Yu and colleagues.[4] The results of this meta-analysis showed that there were statistically significant differences between the omalizumab group and the control group in the following aspects: daily nasal symptom score (standardized mean difference [SMD] = −0.443; 95% confidence interval [CI], −0.538 to −0.347; P<.001); daily ocular symptom score (SMD = −0.385; 95% CI, −0.5 to −0.269; P<.001); daily nasal medication symptom scores (SMD = −0.421; 95% CI, −0.591 to −0.251; P<.001); proportion of days of emergency drug use (risk ratio [RR] = 0.488; 95% CI, 0.307–0.788; P<.005); and rhinoconjunctivitis-specific quality of life questionnaire score (SMD = −0.286; 95% CI, −0.418 to −0.154; P<.001). Importantly, there was no statistically significant difference in safety indicator: adverse events (RR = 1.026; 95% CI, 0.916–1.150; P = .655). The investigators concluded that omalizumab is effective and relatively safe in patients with allergic rhinitis.

Omalizumab has also been studied in patients on allergen immunotherapy. The hypothesis is that neutralization of IgE and reduction of IgE receptor expression on mast cells and basophils could eliminate, or at least reduce the severity of, allergen immunotherapy–related reactions, especially anaphylaxis. In the meta-analysis mentioned earlier, it was noted that omalizumab significantly improved redness and swelling at immunotherapy injection sites. Yu and colleagues[4] concluded that omalizumab used in conjunction with allergen-specific immunotherapy has shown promising results, especially in reducing adverse events.

In a randomized controlled trial, Casale and colleagues[5] evaluated the effectiveness of omalizumab in enhancing both safety and efficacy of rush immunotherapy.[6] Adult patients with ragweed allergic rhinitis were enrolled in a 3-center, 4-arm, double-blind, parallel-group, placebo-controlled trial. Patients received either 9 weeks of omalizumab or placebo, followed by 1-day rush or placebo immunotherapy, then 12 weeks of omalizumab or placebo plus immunotherapy. Patients receiving omalizumab plus rush immunotherapy had fewer adverse events than those receiving immunotherapy alone. The addition of omalizumab resulted in a 5-fold decrease in risk of anaphylaxis caused by rush immunotherapy (odds ratio, 0.17; P = .026).

As noted in the studies described here, omalizumab has been shown to be effective in reducing nasal symptom scores and improving quality of life in several studies of seasonal and perennial allergic rhinitis.[6] However, despite this demonstrated efficacy, omalizumab was not approved by the FDA for the treatment of allergic rhinitis. It was thought that the high cost of omalizumab precluded its chronic use for allergic rhinitis; however, its periodic use may be justified in treatment-resistant patients, especially those with seasonal disease.[7]

Other type 2 biologics have not been studied specifically in allergic rhinitis.

Dupilumab

Dupilumab is a human Ig4 monoclonal antibody directed against the IL-4 receptor subunit α (IL-4Rα), which is recognized by both IL-4 and IL-13. Although dupilumab has not completed studies specifically in allergic rhinitis, studies have assessed the efficacy of dupilumab for the treatment of allergic rhinitis in the setting of comorbid asthma. In patients with uncontrolled persistent asthma despite using medium-dose to high-dose inhaled corticosteroids plus long-acting β2-agonists with comorbid perennial allergic rhinitis, dupilumab's effect on the allergic rhinitis–associated items on the Sino-Nasal Outcome Test (SNOT-22) was studied. In patients with asthma with perennial allergic rhinitis, dupilumab 300 mg every 2 weeks versus placebo significantly improved all 4 allergic rhinitis–associated symptoms of the SNOT-22 (nasal blockage, −0.60; 95% CI, −0.96 to −0.25; runny nose, −0.67; 95% CI, −1.04 to −0.31; sneezing, −0.55; 95% CI, −0.89 to −0.21; postnasal discharge, −0.49; 95% CI, −0.83 to −0.16; all P<.01).[8]

Mepolizumab

Although allergic rhinitis is often thought of as exclusively an IgE-mediated disorder, eosinophilia is a hallmark of this disease process as well. IL-5 is a key mediator acting at many levels of eosinophil biology. Mepolizumab is a humanized anti–IL-5 antibody.

None of the IL-5/IL-5R biologics have been studied specifically in allergic rhinitis. However, a poster presented at the 2019 annual meeting of the American Academy of Allergy, Asthma and Immunology described a meta-analysis of patients with severe asthma from the mepolizumab phase 2b/3 clinical program (DREAM, MENSA, SIRIUS, and MUSCA) with self-reported history of comorbid upper airway disease including allergic rhinitis. Mepolizumab improved quality-of-life assessments in patients with severe asthma and self-reported upper airway disease.[9]

BIOLOGICS FOR ASTHMA

A simplified, streamlined overview of the type 2 inflammatory pathway and the immunologic targets for currently FDA-approved monoclonal agents for the treatment of certain endotypes of asthma is provided in **Fig. 1**. Familiarity with type 2 inflammation is helpful for the practical application because the currently FDA-approved biologic therapies target portions of the type 2 inflammatory cascade.

Recent updates to the Global Initiative for Asthma (GINA) and the European Respiratory Society (ERS)/American Thoracic Society (ATS) guidelines have renewed focus

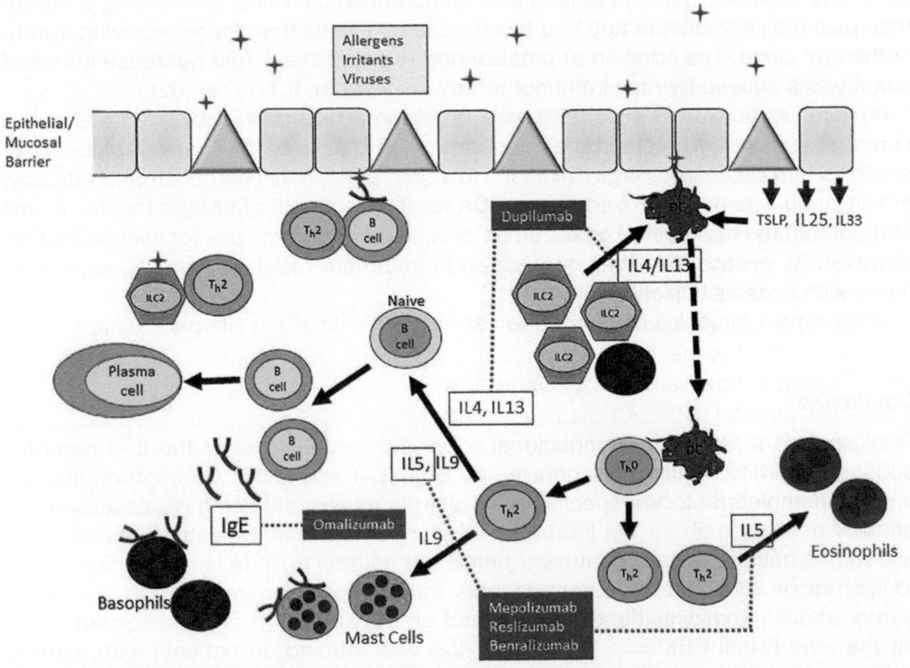

Fig. 1. A general overview of type 2 inflammation. B cell, B lymphocyte; DC, dendritic cell; ILC2, innate type 2 lymphoid cell; Th0, naive T-helper cell; TSLP, thymic stromal lymphopoietin. (*From* Franzese, C. Brief Immunology Review for Targeted Biologic Therapies in Allergic Disease. Curr Otorhinolaryngol Rep 8, 14–18 (2020). https://doi.org/10.1007/s40136-020-00263-0; with permission.)

on treating severe asthma. According to the GINA 2020 update, anti-IgE therapy should be considered as add-on therapy for adolescents, adults, and children (aged 6–11 years) with asthma poorly controlled on moderate-dose inhaled corticosteroids (ICS) and long-acting beta-agonist (LABA) (ie, step 5 treatment).[10] Anti–IL-5/5R therapy should be considered as add-on therapy for adults and adolescents (aged $\geq$12 years), with asthma poorly controlled on medium-dose ICS and LABA (ie, step 5 therapy).[10] There are currently 3 FDA-approved drugs to treat the IL-5 inflammatory pathway: mepolizumab, reslizumab, and benralizumab. Anti–IL-4R therapy should be considered as add-on therapy for adults and adolescents (aged $\geq$12 years) with asthma poorly controlled on moderate-dose ICS and LABA (ie, step 5 therapy).[10]

All but 1 of the following listed biologic agents has an FDA approval for an asthma indication. **Table 1**provides a summary of the pivotal trials supporting the approved asthma indications.

Omalizumab

Omalizumab is a humanized monoclonal antibody that functions as an IgE antagonist, binding to free-floating IgE, specifically to the Cε3 domain; however, cell surface–bound IgE is unaffected.[11,12] Binding of IgE to cell surface receptors depends on exposure to the Cε3 domain. When omalizumab attaches to the Cε3 domain of serum IgE, it inhibits binding to the FcεRI high-affinity IgE receptor and the CD23 receptor.[12] This process diminishes release of inflammatory mediators and upregulates the replacement of FcεRI high-affinity IgE receptors with FcεRII low-affinity IgE receptors.[12] Omalizumab cannot bind to or displace bound IgE because it requires exposure of Cε3 domain and, thus, is unable to bind directly to any IgE receptors itself. In theory, this prevents omalizumab from triggering mediator release and anaphylaxis.

Omalizumab is currently indicated for the treatment of poorly controlled or uncontrolled moderate to severe persistent asthma despite ICS in patients 6 years of age and older with a positive skin test or specific IgE reactivity to a perennial allergen, as add-on maintenance treatment of nasal polyps in patients 18 years of age and older with inadequate response to nasal corticosteroids, and for chronic idiopathic urticaria in patients 12 years of age or older who remain symptomatic despite H1 antihistamine treatment.[13]

Omalizumab is administered via subcutaneous injection and is available as a prefilled syringe or lyophilized powder for reconstitution. Dosage for omalizumab is IgE and weight based. Injection-site pain is the most common adverse reaction seen with omalizumab. Additional warnings include malignancy, helminth infections, and cardiovascular disease, as well as a special black-box warning concerning anaphylaxis. The black-box warning was placed after adverse events were noted in postmarketing, with at least 0.2% of patients who received omalizumab reporting anaphylactic reactions.[14] The Omalizumab Joint Task Force published a report recommending that patients receiving omalizumab be prescribed an autoinjectable form of epinephrine and be observed for 2 hours after the first 3 injections and 30 minutes for all subsequent injections.[15,16]

A higher incidence of malignancies in the omalizumab-treated group compared with the control group (0.5% vs 0.2%) was reported in the initial pooled analysis of phase I and II trials.[17] These malignancies were heterogeneous in tumor type and organ involvement.[18] In the EXCELS observational study, there was no significant difference found in the adjusted malignancy rate in patients treated with omalizumab.[19]

Mepolizumab

Mepolizumab is a humanized monoclonal antibody that functions as an IL-5 antagonist by binding directly to IL-5 and preventing it from binding to the IL-5 receptor α

Table 1
Pivotal trials supporting approved indications for asthma

Biologic Agent	Inclusion Criteria	Effects and Outcomes	Notable Findings
Omalizumab (IgE)	12–75 y old, asthma inadequately controlled with ICS + SPT to DF, DP, cockroach, dog, or cat and total IgE ≥30 IU/mL to 700 IU/mL	Reduced exacerbations (40% overall/60% if eos >300 cells/μL) Improved QOL Decreased ICS use Decreased asthma symptoms	Improved responses with ↑FeNO and eos> 300 cell/μL Improvement in FEV1 less consistent
Reslizumab (IL-5)	18–75 y old, asthma inadequately controlled with ICS + LABA, LTRA, or cromolyn ACQ at 1.5 or more Sputum eosinophils >3%	Reduced exacerbations (approximately 50%–60%) Improved FEV1 (0.100–0.160 L)	Greatest improvement in FEV1 of all 3 anti–IL-5 agents
Mepolizumab (IL-5)	18–82 y old, asthma inadequately controlled with ICS + 1 additional controller ≥2 exacerbations in past year treated with OCS Eosinophils>150 cells/μL at screening; >300 cells/μL within past year	Reduced exacerbations (47%–53% overall/79% if eos >500 cells/μL) Improved FEV1 (0.100 L overall/0.122 L if eos >500 cell/μL)	Most efficacious with eos >500 cell/μL
Benralizumab (IL-5)	12–75 y old, asthma inadequately controlled with ICS + LABA ≥2 exacerbations in past year	Reduced exacerbations (28%–51%) Improved FEV1 (0.100–0.160 L)	Efficacy correlates with increased eos
Dupilumab (IL-4/13)	>18 y old, asthma inadequately controlled on medium to high dose with ICS + LABA ≥ 1 exacerbation in past year	Reduced exacerbations (60%–80%) Improved FEV1 (0.150–0.160 L)	Most effective if eos> 300 cell/μL

Abbreviations: +, positive; ACQ, asthma control questionnaire; DF, *Dermatophagoides farinae*; DP, *Dermatophagoides pteronyssinus*; eos, eosinophils; FeNO, fractional exhaled nitric oxide; FEV1, forced expiratory volume in 1 second; LABA, long-acting beta-agonist; LTRA, leukotriene receptor antagonist; OCS, oral corticosteroids;QOL, quality of life; SPT, skin prick test.

From Damask CC, Ryan MW, Casale TB, et al. Targeted Molecular Therapies in Allergy and Rhinology. Otolaryngology–Head and Neck Surgery. 2021;164(1_suppl): S1-S21. https://doi.org/10.1177/0194599820965233; with permissions per STM Permissions Guidelines.

subunit. It is currently indicated as add-on maintenance therapy for the treatment of patients with poorly controlled or uncontrolled severe asthma with an eosinophilic phenotype aged 6 years and older, patients aged 18 years or older with eosinophilic granulomatosis with polyangiitis (EGPA), and for treatment of patients aged 12 years and older with hypereosinophilic syndrome (HES) for greater than or equal to 6 months without an identifiable nonhematologic secondary cause.[20]

Because subjects in the mepolizumab trials had peripheral eosinophil counts greater than 150 cells/μL, this is often the minimum requirement from insurance companies for coverage. Mepolizumab is administered subcutaneously every 4 weeks with a dose of 40 mg for patients aged 6 years to 11 years and 100 mg for patients more than 12 years of age.[20] Its dosage is not weight based. Mepolizumab is available in a lyophilized powder that has to be reconstituted for administration in a health care setting and in a prefilled syringe form as well as an autoinjector, both for home administration. In the clinical trials, 2 mepolizumab-treated subjects and none of the placebo-treated subjects developed shingles in studies of more than 1300 subjects. The label states that clinicians should consider varicella vaccination in patients in whom such protection is medically appropriate before starting mepolizumab. The label also recommends treating patients with preexisting helminth infections before therapy with mepolizumab.[20]

Reslizumab

Reslizumab is also a humanized monoclonal antibody that functions as an IL-5 antagonist by binding directly to IL-5 and preventing its binding to the IL-5 receptor α subunit. It is currently indicated as add-on maintenance therapy for adult patients with poorly or uncontrolled severe asthma with an eosinophilic phenotype.[21]

Subjects in the reslizumab trials had peripheral eosinophil counts greater than 400 cells/μL; insurance companies often require levels greater than this for approval. Reslizumab's dosing is weight based at 3 mg/kg once every 4 weeks administered by intravenous infusion over 20 to 50 minutes, making it a good option for obese patients. Anaphylaxis was observed with reslizumab infusion in 0.3% of patients in placebo-controlled clinical studies. Anaphylaxis was reported as early as the second dose.[22] Also, 0.6% of patients in placebo-controlled clinical studies had at least 1 malignant neoplasm reported compared with 0.3% of patients in the placebo group. The observed malignancies in reslizumab-treated patients were diverse and without clustering of any particular tissue type.[21]

Benralizumab

Benralizumab is a humanized monoclonal antibody that is specifically engineered without a fucose molecule and binds directly to the IL-5 receptor α subunit.[23] When bound, it can trigger antibody-dependent cell cytotoxicity and apoptosis in eosinophils and mast cells.[23] Although benralizumab is in essence an IL-5 antagonist, its mechanism of action is technically different from mepolizumab and reslizumab, because it induces eosinophilic cell death, as opposed to binding to IL-5 itself. It is currently indicated as add-on maintenance therapy for the treatment of patients with poorly controlled or uncontrolled severe asthma with an eosinophilic phenotype aged 12 years and older.[23] It was also granted orphan drug status for adult patients with EGPA in November 2018, for hypereosinophilic syndrome (HES) in February 2019, and eosinophilic esophagitis in August 2019.[24]

Benralizumab is administered subcutaneously every 4 weeks with a fixed dose of 30 mg for patients aged 12 years of age and older for the initial 3 doses, then administered every 8 weeks thereafter. Given that, after the first 3 doses, the dosing interval is expanded to almost 2 months, this results in fewer injections and may be more convenient for some patients with transportation difficulties or other lifestyle barriers. Similar to mepolizumab, benralizumab's dosing is not weight based. Benralizumab is available as a prefilled syringe for home administration or administration in a health care setting, as well as an autoinjector for home administration. Patients with preexisting helminth infections need to be treated before initiating therapy with benralizumab.[23]

Dupilumab

Dupilumab is a fully human monoclonal antibody that functions as an IL-4 receptor α-subunit antagonist. Although this agent only binds to the IL-4 receptor α subunit, it inhibits the signaling of both IL-4 and IL-13 because this particular subunit is present in both type I receptors, which bind IL-4, and type II receptors, which bind IL-4 and IL-13. It is currently approved as an add-on maintenance treatment in patients aged 18 years or older with inadequately controlled chronic rhinosinusitis with nasal polyposis, as well as the treatment of patients aged 6 years or older with moderate to severe atopic dermatitis uncontrolled by topical treatments, and as an add-on maintenance treatment in patients with moderate to severe asthma aged 12 years and older with eosinophilic phenotype and/or oral corticosteroid (OCS)-dependent asthma.[25]

In adults and adolescents (12 years of age and older) for moderate to severe asthma, an initial dose of 400 mg (2 200-mg injections) followed by 200 mg given every other week, or an initial dose of 600 mg (2 300-mg injections) followed by 300 mg given every other week, is administered subcutaneously either in a health care setting or at home via a prefilled syringe (for 200-mg and 300-mg options) or a prefilled pen (for 300 mg only). For patients requiring concomitant OCS or with comorbid moderate to severe atopic dermatitis, for which dupilumab is indicated, it is recommended to start with an initial dose of 600 mg followed by 300 mg given every other week.[25]

In the atopic dermatitis trials, dupilumab was associated with a higher incidence of conjunctivitis compared with subjects receiving placebo.[26] Dupilumab-treated subjects in the nasal polyp trials had a greater initial increase from baseline in blood eosinophil count compared with subjects treated with placebo, which is likely related to its underlying mechanism of action in blocking IL-4–mediated eosinophil migration out of the bloodstream.[27] Because the clinical significance of the transient increase in eosinophil level is unknown, it is recommended that clinicians be alert to vasculitic rash, worsening pulmonary symptoms, and/or neuropathy, especially on reduction of OCS.

Tezepelumab

Tezepelumab is a subcutaneously administered humanized monoclonal antibody that blocks the action of thymic stromal lymphopoietin (TSLP), an epithelial cytokine.[28,29] TSLP sits at the top of multiple inflammatory cascades and plays a critical role in the initiation and persistence of allergic, eosinophilic, and other types of airway inflammation associated with severe asthma. TSLP is released in response to multiple triggers, including allergens, viruses, and other airborne particles, associated with asthma exacerbations. Blocking TSLP may prevent the release of proinflammatory cytokines by immune cells, resulting in the prevention of asthma exacerbations and improved asthma control.[30]

NAVIGATOR is a phase III, randomized, double-blinded, placebo-controlled trial in adults and adolescents (aged $\geq$12 years) with severe uncontrolled asthma who were receiving treatment with medium-dose or high-dose ICS plus at least 1 additional controller medicine with or without OCS. NAVIGATOR met the primary end point with tezepelumab added to standard of care, showing a statistically significant and clinically meaningful reduction in the annualized asthma exacerbation rate over 52 weeks compared with placebo.[31–33]

SOURCE is a phase III, multicenter, randomized, double-blinded, parallel-group, placebo-controlled trial for 48 weeks in adult patients with severe asthma who require continuous treatment with ICS plus LABA, and chronic treatment with maintenance OCS therapy. Patients were randomized to receive tezepelumab every 4 weeks or placebo as add-on therapy.[34] However, the SOURCE trial did not meet the primary end point of a statistically significant reduction in the daily OCS dose, without loss of asthma control, with tezepelumab compared with placebo.[35]

FUTURE DIRECTIONS

As additional trials continue for new biologic agents for asthma, an interesting shift seems to be occurring among potential biologic treatments for allergic rhinitis. Although cytokine-based or anti-IgE–based biologics seem to be helpful as add-on therapy to other treatments, none of them have been resoundingly successful as solo treatments for allergic rhinitis. Perhaps because of this, there has been interest in and development of monoclonal antibodies targeting specific epitopes on certain common allergens, such as cat and birch tree pollen.[36,37] Some of these trials involve investigating a single dosing treatment to a sustain an entire allergy season or whether there is blocking activity preventing symptomatic experience of pollen-food syndrome.[37] Whether any of these epitope-targeting monoclonal antibodies show efficacy remains to be seen, but their development opens up exciting possibilities for future treatment strategies.

SUMMARY

At present, monoclonal antibodies targeting type 2 inflammation are primarily indicated as add-on treatment to standard of care, maintenance therapy for patients with asthma and other approved disorders. However, because these agents target cytokines and cell surface receptors integral to type 2 inflammation, which is the underlying type of inflammation shared by several disease processes, they have the potential to treat more than 1 disorder and may change how patient care for atopic disorders is managed. Knowledge of the type 2 immunologic cascade will prove useful to agent selection, but practical matters such as frequency of injection, location (home vs office) of injection, weight based or not, and method (subcutaneous vs intravenous) of administration are important considerations as well.

CLINICS CARE POINTS

- Biologic therapies are add-ons to standard-of-care treatments. Ensuring patients have tried and been compliant with such therapy before starting a biologic agent is important.
- Dosing, route, and frequency of administration vary between different agents. Treating practitioners should consider these aspects when selecting a therapy.
- Patients who have not had the varicella vaccination may be at risk for shingles. Depending on the agent selected, a discussion with the patient regarding risks or consideration for a shingles vaccination may be necessary.

DISCLOSURE

No funding was provided for this article. These are conflicts of interest. C. Franzese: speakers bureau for ALK, GSK, Regeneron, Sanofi, Optinose, AstraZeneca; advisory board for ALK, GSK, Genentech; research support for ALK, Novartis, Shiniogi, Bellus, Merck, Genentech, Regeneron. C. Damask: advisory board for ALK, GSK, Genentech, Sanofi; consultant for AstraZeneca, Audigy Medical, Novartis; research support for AstraZeneca, GSK, OptiNose; speakers bureau for AstraZeneca, GSK, OptiNose, Regeneron, Sanofi.

REFERENCES

1. Shamji MH, Durham SR. Mechanisms of allergen immunotherapy for inhaled allergens and predictive biomarkers. J Allergy Clin Immunol 2017;140:1485–98.
2. Gandhi NA, Bennett BL, Graham NMH, et al. Targeting key proximal drivers of type 2 inflammation in disease. Nat Rev Drug Discov 2016;15(1):35–40.
3. Stevens WW, Peters AT, Tan BK, et al. Associations between inflammatory endotypes and clinical presentations in Chronic Rhinosinusitis. J Allergy Clin Immunol Pract 2019;7(8):2812–20.e3.
4. Yu C, Wang K, Cui X, et al. Clinical efficacy and safety of omalizumab in the treatment of allergic rhinitis: a systematic review and meta-analysis of randomized clinical trials. Am J Rhinol Allergy 2020;34(2):196–208.
5. Casale TB, Busse WW, Kline JN, et al, Immune Tolerance Network Group. Omalizumab pretreatment decreases acute reactions after rush immunotherapy for ragweed-induced seasonal allergic rhinitis. J Allergy Clin Immunol 2006;117(1):134–40.
6. Polk P, Stokes J. Anti-IgE therapy. In: Cox LS, editor. Immunotherapies for allergic disease. 1. Philadelphia: Elsevier Health Sciences; 2019. p. 355–72.
7. Vashisht P, Casale T. Omalizumab for treatment of allergic rhinitis. Expert Opin Biol Ther 2013;13(6):933–45.
8. Weinstein SF, Katial R, Jayawardena S, et al. Efficacy and safety of dupilumab in perennial allergic rhinitis and comorbid asthma. J Allergy Clin Immunol 2018;142(1):171–7.e1.
9. Prazma CM, Albers F, Mallett S, et al. Poster 283: Mepolizumab improves patient outcomes and reduces exacerbations in severe asthma patients with comorbid upper airways disease. Available at: https://aaaai.confex.com/aaaai/2019/webprogram/Paper40909.html. Accessed December 24, 2020.
10. Global initiative for asthma global strategy for management and prevention 2020 update. Available at: https://ginasthma.org/gina-reports. Accessed December 25, 2020.
11. Damask CC. Biologics. In: Franzese CB, Damask CC, Wise SK, et al, editors. Handbook of otolaryngic allergy. New York: Thieme; 2019.
12. Johansson SGO, Haahtela T, O'Byrne M. Omalizumab and the immune system: an overview of preclinical and clinical data. Ann Allergy Asthma Immunol 2002;89:132–8.
13. Omalizumab package insert. Available at: https://www.gene.com/download/pdf/xolair_prescribing.pdf. Accessed December 7, 2020.
14. Limb SL, Starke PR, Lee CE, et al. Delayed onset and protracted progression of anaphylaxis after omalizumab administration in patients with asthma. J Allergy Clin Immunol 2007;120(6):1378–81.
15. Cox L, Platts-Mills TA, Finegold I, et al. American Academy of Allergy, Asthma & Immunology/American College of Allergy, Asthma and Immunology Joint Task Force Report on omalizumab-associated anaphylaxis. J Allergy Clin Immunol 2007;120(6):1373–7.

16. Cox L, Lieberman P, Wallace D, et al. American Academy of Allergy, Asthma & Immunology/American College of Allergy, Asthma & Immunology Omalizumab Associated Anaphylaxis Joint Task Force follow-up report. J Allergy Clin Immunol 2011;128(1):210–2.
17. Xolair (Omalizumab) for Subcutaneous Use—Genentech, Inc.. 2008. Available at: http://www.xolair.com/prescribing_information.html. Accessed December 7, 2020.
18. Data on file. Genentech and Novartis Pharmaceuticals Corporation; 2008. Available at: https://nam03.safelinks.protection.outlook.com/?url=https%3A%2F%2Fwww.xolairhcp.com%2Fcontent%2Fdam%2Fgene%2Fxolairhcp%2Fpdfs%2FXOLAIR-Nasal-Polyps-PI-Visual-Aid.pi.pdf%3Fnocache%3Dtrue&data=04%7C01%7Cj.surendrakumar%40elsevier.com%7Cef1abd6a42954fb1328b08d91f80d263%7C9274ee3f94254109a27f9fb15c10675d%7C0%7C0%7C637575461069470862%7CUnknown%7CTWFpbGZsb3d8eyJWIjoiMC4wLjAwMDAiLCJQIjoiV2luMzIiLCJBTiI6Ik1haWwiLCJXVCI6Mn0%3D%7C1000&sdata=AhFT4ByurromHmRFtv5BgL55YrTV2MnNF%2FCt5UX9fF0%3D&reserved=0 accessed 5/24/21. Referenced can be changed to https://nam03.safelinks.protection.outlook.com/?url=https%3A%2F%2Fwww.xolairhcp.-com%2Fcontent%2Fdam%2Fgene%2Fxolairhcp%2Fpdfs%2FXOLAIR-Nasal-Polyps-PI-Visual-Aid.pi.pdf%3Fnocache%3Dtrue&data=04%7C01%7Cj.surendrakumar%40elsevier.com%7Cef1abd6a42954fb1328b08d91f80d263%7C9274ee3f94254109a27f9fb15c10675d%7C0%7C0%7C637575461069470862%7CUnknown%7CTWFpbGZsb3d8eyJWIjoiMC4wLjAwMDAiLCJQIjoiV2luMzIiLCJBTiI6Ik1haWwiLCJXVCI6Mn0%3D%7C1000&sdata=AhFT4ByurromHmRFtv5BgL55YrTV2MnNF%2FCt5UX9fF0%3D&reserved=0. Accessed May 24, 2021.
19. Janson SL, Solari PG, Trzaskoma B, et al. Omalizumab adherence in an observational study of patients with moderate to severe allergic asthma. Ann Allergy Asthma Immunol 2015;114(6):516–21.
20. Mepolizumab package insert. Available at: https://gsksource.com/pharma/content/dam/GlaxoSmithKline/US/en/Prescribing_Information/Nucala/pdf/NUCALA-PI-PIL-IFU-COMBINED.PDF. Accessed December 7, 2020.
21. Reslizumab package insert. Available at: https://www.cinqair.com/globalassets/cinqair/prescribinginformation.pdf. Accessed December 7, 2020.
22. Castro M, Zangrilli J, Wechsler ME, et al. Reslizumab for inadequately controlled asthma with elevated blood eosinophil counts: results from two multicentre, parallel, double-blind, randomised, placebo-controlled, phase 3 trials. Lancet Respir Med. 2015 May;3(5):355-366. doi: 10.1016/S2213-2600(15)00042-9. Epub 2015 Feb 23. Erratum in: Lancet Respir Med. 2015 Apr;3(4):e15. Erratum in: Lancet Respir Med. Lancet Respir Med 2016;4(10):e50.
23. Benralizumab package insert. Available at: https://www.azpicentral.com/fasenra/fasenra.pdf#page=1. Accessed December 7, 2020.
24. Benralizumab Receives Orphan Drug Status for Eosinophilic Esophagitis. Available at: https://www.empr.com/home/news/drugs-in-the-pipeline/benralizumab-receives-orphan-drug-status-for-eosinophilic-esophagitis/. Accessed December 7, 2020.
25. Dupilumab package insert. Available at: https://www.regeneron.com/sites/default/files/Dupixent_FPI.pdf. Accessed December 7, 2020.
26. Simpson EL, Bieber T, Guttman-Yassky E, et al, SOLO 1 and SOLO 2 Investigators. Two phase 3 trials of dupilumab versus placebo in atopic dermatitis. N Engl J Med 2016;375(24):2335–48.

27. Damask CC, Ryan MW, Casale TB, et al. Targeted molecular therapies in allergy and rhinology. Otolaryngol Head Neck Surg 2020;3. https://doi.org/10.1177/0194599820965233. 194599820965233.
28. Varricchi G, Pecoraro A, Marone G, et al. Thymic stromal lymphopoietin isoforms, inflammatory disorders, and cancer. Front Immunol 2018;9:1595.
29. Corren J, Parnes JR, Wang L, et al. Tezepelumab in adults with uncontrolled asthma [published correction appears in N Engl J Med. 2019 May 23; 380 (21): 2082]. N Engl J Med 2017;377(10):936–46.
30. Li Y, Wang W, Lv Z, et al. Elevated expression of IL-33 and TSLP in the airways of human asthmatics in vivo: a potential biomarker of severe refractory disease. J Immunol 2018;200:2253–62.
31. Clinicaltrials.gov. Study to evaluate tezepelumab in adults & adolescents with severe uncontrolled asthma (NAVIGATOR). Available at: https://clinicaltrials.gov/ct2/show/NCT03347279. Accessed December 25, 2020.
32. Menzies-Gow A, Colice G, Griffiths JM, et al. NAVIGATOR: a phase 3 multicentre, randomized, double-blind, placebo-controlled, parallel-group trial to evaluate the efficacy and safety of tezepelumab in adults and adolescents with severe, uncontrolled asthma. Respir Res 2020;21(1):266.
33. AstraZeneca plc. Tezepelumab NAVIGATOR Phase III trial met primary endpoint of a statistically significant and clinically meaningful reduction in exacerbations in a broad population of patients with severe asthma. Available at: https://www.astrazeneca.com/content/astraz/media-centre/press-releases/2020/tezepelumab-navigator-phase-iii-trial-met-primary-endpoint.html. Accessed December 25, 2020.
34. Wechsler ME, Colice G, Griffiths JM, et al. SOURCE: a phase 3, multicentre, randomized, double-blind, placebo-controlled, parallel group trial to evaluate the efficacy and safety of tezepelumab in reducing oral corticosteroid use in adults with oral corticosteroid dependent asthma. Respir Res 2020;21:264.
35. Update on SOURCE Phase III trial for tezepelumab in patients with severe, oral corticosteroid-dependent asthma. Available at: https://www.astrazeneca.com/media-centre/press-releases/2020/update-on-source-phase-iii-trial-for-tezepelumab-in-patients-with-severe-oral-corticosteroid-dependent-asthma.html. Accessed December 25, 2020.
36. Orengo JM, Radin AR, Kamat V, et al. Treating cat allergy with monoclonal IgG antibodies that bind allergen and prevent IgE engagement. Nat Commun 2018; 9(1):1421.
37. Atanasio A, Franklin M, Ben LH, et al. Targeting birch allergy with monoclonal IgG antibodies that bind allergen and prevent IgE effector cell activation. J Allergy Clin Immunol 2020;9(1):1421. Available at: https://www.jacionline.org/article/S0091-6749(19)32421-2/pdf.

Immunotherapeutic Strategies for Head and Neck Cancer

Zachary S. Buchwald, MD, PhD[a,b], Nicole C. Schmitt, MD[c,*]

KEYWORDS

• Biologics • Monoclonal antibodies • Immunotherapy • Otolaryngology • Cancer
• PD-1

KEY POINTS

- Immunotherapy for head and neck squamous cell carcinoma (HNSCC) consists primarily of biologic agents, including monoclonal antibodies, vaccines, and whole immune cells.
- Inhibitors of the programmed cell death protein 1 (PD-1) immune checkpoint pathway are in use for recurrent/metastatic HNSCC and are currently under investigation for previously untreated, locally advanced disease.
- Preventive vaccines for human papilloma virus (HPV) are not useful for treatment of pre-existing HPV-related oropharyngeal carcinoma, but several therapeutic vaccines for HPV-related HNSCC are in development.
- Combinations of immunotherapy with chemotherapy, radiation, or surgery have shown encouraging results in HNSCC. The combination of anti–PD-1 therapy plus cytotoxic chemotherapy has been US Food and Drug Administration approved for recurrent/metastatic disease.

INTRODUCTION

Surgery, radiation, and cytotoxic chemotherapy have been used for decades to treat head and neck squamous cell carcinoma (HNSCC). In recent decades, immunotherapy has revolutionized the treatment of cancer, including HNSCC. Most immune therapies consist of biologics, including monoclonal antibodies, vaccines, and cell therapy. This article reviews basic tumor immunology, then provides an overview of immunotherapeutic strategies in use and under investigation for HNSCC. For further

[a] Winship Cancer Institute, Emory University School of Medicine, 1365 Clifton Road NE, C5086, Atlanta, GA 30322, USA; [b] Department of Radiation Oncology, Emory University School of Medicine, Atlanta, GA, USA; [c] Department of Otolaryngology – Head and Neck Surgery, Emory University School of Medicine, Atlanta, GA, USA
* Corresponding author. Head and Neck Cancer Program, Winship Cancer Institute, Emory University School of Medicine, 550 Peachtree Street Northeast, 11th Floor Otolaryngology, Atlanta, GA 30308.
E-mail address: nicole.cherie.schmitt@emory.edu

Otolaryngol Clin N Am 54 (2021) 729–742
https://doi.org/10.1016/j.otc.2021.04.004
oto.theclinics.com

information, some of these strategies are covered in more detail elsewhere in this issue.

DISCUSSION

Basics of Tumor Immunology and Immunotherapy

Cancer can be viewed as a genetic disorder in which cellular stress/inflammation induced by carcinogens (eg, tobacco) leads to genomic instability and impaired ability to undergo cell death. Innate and adaptive immunity exist, in part, to eliminate nascent malignant cells. However, clinically significant tumors evolve ways, under the harsh selective pressure of the immune system, to escape and thrive.

The innate immune system is the first line of defense against the stress signals that lead to tumor formation. Stressed, inflamed cells release damage-associated molecular patterns (DAMPs),[1] which result in the trafficking of immune cells into the tumor milieu. Natural killer (NK) cells recognize and kill cells that show generic stress signals. Innate immunity is a rapid, nonspecific response. In contrast, adaptive immunity is antigen specific and durable. In general, for a robust adaptive immune response, tumor neoantigens, proteins perceived as foreign that can be recognized by antigen-specific T cells, are required. In HNSCC, these antigens can consist of proteins that are expressed at high levels (eg, epidermal growth factor receptor), mutated proteins (eg, p53), or viral material, such as human papillomavirus (HPV) oncoproteins. In order for these neoantigens to be presented to a T cell, they must first be processed inside the cell, loaded onto a major histocompatibility complex (MHC; also known as human leukocyte antigen [HLA]) molecule in the endoplasmic reticulum, then shuttled to the surface of the cell. The peptide-MHC complex is then bound by antigen-specific T-cell receptors (TCRs; **Fig. 1**). For antigen-presenting cells such as dendritic cells, antigen processing and presentation is a full-time job. These cells engulf proteins found in the environment, process the material, and present potential antigens to T cells. Once the TCR is linked to a peptide-MHC complex, activation of costimulatory receptors (CD28) is an important second signal for T-cell activation. The third important signal is production of cytokines, which leads to T-cell proliferation and differentiation.

However, cancer cells have evolved numerous ways of escaping under the selective pressure of the immune system. Tumor cells can adapt to express fewer neoantigens over time, a process known as immunoediting. Tumor cells that do express neoantigens can downregulate expression of MHC-I and other cellular components needed for antigen processing and presentation to immune cells. Even if neoantigens are present and properly processed, immune cells must be present to respond to them; tumors that exclude immune effectors (said to be immunologically cold) or are heavily infiltrated by immunosuppressive cells may also escape immune surveillance. In addition, the expression of coinhibitory checkpoints, such as programmed cell death 1 (PD-1) on T cells and its ligand PD-L1 on tumor and other tumor infiltrating cells, also inhibits antitumor immunity (**Fig. 2**). The evolved purpose of coinhibitory checkpoints is to prevent exaggerated immune responses (eg, autoimmunity), but cancer cells can exploit this system by expressing high levels of PD-L1 to avoid killing by T cells.

Most immunotherapeutic treatments work by enhancing the action of immune effector cells ("stepping on the gas") or by inhibiting these mechanisms of immune escape ("releasing the brakes"; **Table 1**). Combination therapies may use both strategies at once. For example, radiation and cytotoxic chemotherapy preferentially kill cancer cells, releasing antigens and DAMPs, and creating an inflammatory response;

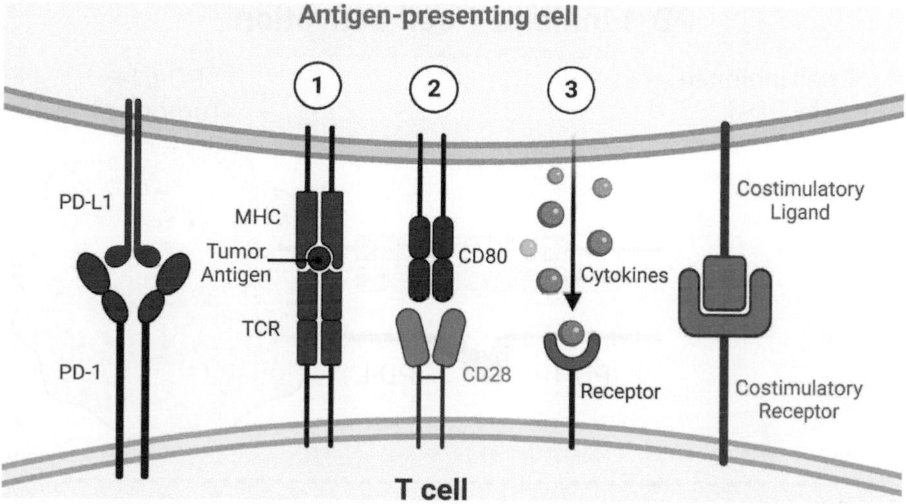

Fig. 1. Three steps are required for initiation of a T-cell response. First, interaction of the TCR with an antigen-MHC complex induces T-cell stimulation (1). Next, interaction of cluster of differentiation (CD) 28 and CD80 leads to T-cell activation (2). In addition, production of cytokines by the antigen-presenting cell (3) leads to T-cell proliferation and differentiation. Interaction of coinhibitory receptors (eg, programmed cell death 1 [PD-1]; *red*) with their ligands (eg, PD-L1) inhibit the T-cell response, whereas the interaction of costimulatory receptors (eg, CD40, CD137, OX40) with their ligands (*green*) promote the T cell response. Created with BioRender.com.

the activity of responding immune cells can then be further enhanced by inhibiting checkpoints such as PD-1. Specific therapeutic strategies are detailed further in the rest of this article and elsewhere in this issue.

Immunotherapeutic Strategies for the Treatment of Head and Neck Cancer

Tumor antigen-targeted monoclonal antibodies

Cetuximab is a chimeric mouse-human immunoglobulin (Ig) G1 monoclonal antibody targeting epidermal growth factor receptor (EGFR), which is overexpressed in most HNSCCs. Cetuximab is US Food and Drug Administration (FDA) approved in combination with radiation for previously untreated disease; this combination is primarily used in cisplatin-ineligible patients. It is also approved as monotherapy or in combination with cytotoxic chemotherapy (cisplatin/fluorouracil) for recurrent or metastatic disease.[2,3] Interestingly, only a subset of patients respond well to cetuximab, and its mechanisms of action are thought to be related to enhanced antitumor immunity rather than EGFR inhibition.[4,5] In support of this idea, tumor antigen-specific T cells correlate with responses to cetuximab in HNSCC.[6,7] The mechanisms of action and indications for cetuximab are further reviewed by Trivedi and Ferris in Epidermal Growth Factor Receptor Targeted Therapy for Head and Neck Cancer.

Immune checkpoints

Coinhibitory checkpoint pathways exist to prevent exaggerated immune responses, but, as noted earlier, tumor cells may exploit these pathways as a mechanism of immune escape. Although several different coinhibitory checkpoints have been identified and studied, PD-1 and cytotoxic T lymphocyte–associated protein 4 (CTLA-4) pathways have been most widely studied thus far. Monoclonal antibodies blocking these

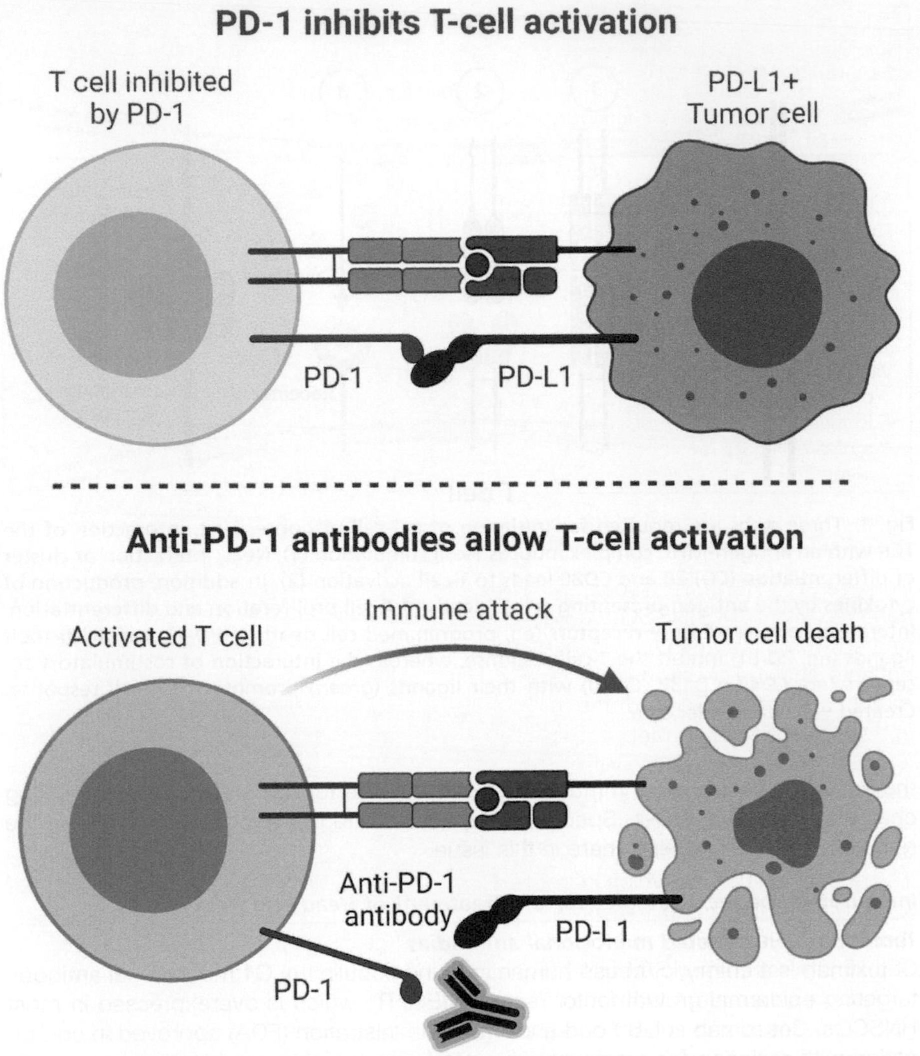

Fig. 2. The interaction of PD-1 on a T cell with its ligand (PD-L1) on a tumor cell inhibits T-cell activation. T-cell activation can be restored by blocking this interaction with anti–PD-1 or anti–PD-L1 antibodies, leading to T-cell killing of the tumor cell. Created with BioRender.com.

pathways have shown encouraging results, first in melanoma, and more recently in HNSCC and other solid tumors.

Programmed cell death 1 pathway. The best-studied immune checkpoint pathway thus far for HNSCC is the PD-1 pathway. Multiple monoclonal antibodies targeting PD-1 or its ligand, PD-L1, are now available. Two PD-1 inhibitors, pembrolizumab and nivolumab, are currently approved for use in recurrent/metastatic (R/M) HNSCC. The standard first-line therapy for R/M HNSCC was the EXTREME regimen, which includes cisplatin, fluorouracil and cetuximab. Approximately one-third of patients respond to the EXTREME regimen, with a median overall survival of 10 months.[8]

Table 1
Immunotherapeutic strategies and current phase of study for head and neck squamous cell carcinoma

Enhancement of Immune Effector Cells (Stepping on the Gas)		Overcoming Immune Escape Mechanisms (Releasing the Brakes)	
Strategy	**Phase of Study**	**Strategy**	**Phase of Study**
Tumor antigen-targeting antibodies (cetuximab)	FDA approved	Checkpoint inhibitors (anti–PD-1/PD-L1)	FDA approved
Costimulatory agonists	Early phase	Inhibition of immunosuppressive cells (MDSCs, Tregs)	Early phase
Vaccines (peptides, viral or bacterial vector)	Early phase	—	
Adoptive cell therapy	Early phase		
Agonists of innate immunity	Early phase		

Abbreviations: FDA, US Food and Drug Administration; MDSCs, myeloid-derived suppressor cells.

However, EXTREME is associated with significant toxicity. In the KEYNOTE-012 trial, patients with R/M HNSCC who had failed first-line, platinum-based therapy were treated with the anti–PD-1 antibody pembrolizumab.[9,10] About a third of the enrolled patients showed a response or stable disease, despite having failed multiple prior rounds of therapy. Some of the responses were durable, often lasting up to 2 years. In the first phase III, randomized, placebo-controlled trial of PD-1 therapy for HNSCC (CheckMate-041), patients with R/M disease who had failed platinum chemotherapy were randomized to receive the anti–PD-1 antibody nivolumab or investigator's choice of second-line therapy (other forms of cytotoxic chemotherapy or cetuximab monotherapy). The trial was stopped early after meeting its primary end point of increased 1-year overall survival, which increased from 17% with standard second-line therapy to 36% with nivolumab.[11] Both anti–PD-1 antibodies were very well tolerated, and these 2 trials led to FDA approval of pembrolizumab and nivolumab for the treatment of platinum-refractory, R/M HNSCC in 2016.

Multiple subsequent trials with PD-1 inhibitors have followed, with similar results: good responses in a subset of patients and stable disease in others, despite failing multiple prior lines of therapy, and a favorable toxicity profile.[12,13] The consistent finding of responses in a minority of patients has sparked tremendous interest in finding biomarkers of response and resistance (see the review by Maroun and Mandal, "Anti-PD-1 immune checkpoint blockade for head and neck cancer: Biomarkers of response and resistance", in this issue). The one predictive biomarker already in wide clinical use is tumor expression of PD-L1.[10,14] The combined positive score (CPS) is the number of PD-L1–positive cells (lymphocytes, macrophages, tumor cells) divided by the total number of viable tumor cells, then multiplied by 100. The CPS was established in order to standardize the assessment of PD-L1 staining for prediction of responses.[12] Although it has been suggested that HPV-related tumors may be more likely to respond to PD-1 inhibition versus HPV-negative tumors, results from clinical trials have been mixed.[9,14–17]

Other coinhibitory and costimulatory receptors. Inhibitors of CTLA-4 are approved for use in melanoma[18] but have shown disappointing results for HNSCC.[19] Multiple preclinical mouse model studies have shown an encouraging rationale for the use of antibodies blocking other coinhibitory checkpoints, including TIM-3, LAG-3, and TIGIT, in addition to PD-1.[20–26]

Rather than release the brakes by targeting coinhibitory receptors, 1 way of stepping on the gas is to enhance T-cell function by activating costimulatory receptors, such as OX40, CD137 (also known as 4-1BB), or CD40. This strategy has been tested in multiple preclinical mouse model studies, and multiple early-phase clinical trials of costimulatory agonists are underway for solid tumors, including HNSCC.[27–29]

Vaccines and oncolytic viruses

Vaccination is the process of introducing a specific antigen or antigens to the immune system with the intent of developing a durable, antigen-specific immune response. Tumor vaccines can be made from peptides, DNA, whole tumor cells, or antigen-presenting cells loaded with a specific tumor antigen. Tumor vaccines can also be delivered by viral or bacterial vectors. The presence of viral antigens in HPV-related disease is a strong rationale for the development of vaccines and other antigen-specific immune therapies for HPV-driven tumors. Preventive vaccines are highly effective for prevention of future HPV infection but not useful for treating established HPV-associated tumors. Several therapeutic vaccines have been developed for cervical cancer and other HPV-related malignancies. However, vaccines consisting of E6, E7, p16^{INK4A}, or other HPV-16 peptides have shown modest results so far.[30–33] Vaccines using viral or bacterial vectors to deliver HPV-specific antigens have also been studied. Multiple early-phase trials using a *Listeria*-based HPV-16 antigen vaccine (ADXS11-001) are enrolling patients with oropharyngeal cancer and other HPV-related cancers.[31,34]

Oncolytic viruses preferentially infect and lyse tumor cells more than normal cells, subsequently releasing tumor antigens from dying cells to the tumor microenvironment where they can be recognized by immune cells.[35] Clinical trials with the T-VEC vaccine (an HSV-1 virus) and other oncolytic viruses for melanoma, HNSCC, and other solid tumors have shown encouraging results.[36–38]

Adoptive cell therapy

Another way to step on the gas is by administering immune effector cells, which is known as adoptive cell transfer. Most commonly, this involves the use of CD8+ T cells, which can be isolated from patients, expanded ex vivo, and then reinfused into the patient. Modifications are often made to make the T cells more effective before expansion and reinfusion. Thus far, most clinical trials involving T-cell transfer in HNSCC have focused on HPV-related disease[39,40] (see the comprehensive overview of adoptive T-cell therapy for HNSCC by Norberg and Hinrichs, in this issue).

However, some tumors do not respond to adoptive transfer of T cells because of a lack of neoantigens or the machinery required to process and present these antigens. These limitations might be overcome by using NK cells or chimeric antigen receptor (CAR) T cells instead. NK cells do not react to specific antigens and do not need to be HLA matched to the host. CARs are artificial TCRs that are engineered to recognize specific antigens and also contain T-cell activation domains. For example, CAR T cells have been engineered to express receptors for ErbB dimers, which are often upregulated in HNSCC, and the 4ab receptor, which converts IL-4 into a signal for T-cell expansion.[41] The use of off-the-shelf NK cell or CAR T-cell products offers attractive strategies that are currently in early-phase clinical trials.[41,42]

Agonists of innate immunity

Toll-like receptors (TLRs) play an important role in the antiviral immune responses, inflammation, and innate/adaptive immunity.[43] TLR agonists act, in part, by maturing antigen-presenting cells to present antigen in an inflammatory context to T cells. In mouse models of HNSCC, agonists of TLR7, TLR8, and TLR9 have shown additive or synergistic activity when combined with cetuximab or PD-1 antibodies.[44–46] A phase 1b trial of a TLR8 agonist (motolimod) combined with cetuximab for R/M HNSCC showed some partial responses and enhanced NK cell activation,[47] but another trial comparing motolimod versus placebo combined with the EXTREME regimen showed no difference in survival.[48] A phase 1b/2 study combining intratumoral injection of a TLR9 agonist (SD-101) with pembrolizumab for R/M HNSCC showed an encouraging disease control rate of 48%.[49]

Type 1 interferons are produced following activation of a protein called stimulator of interferon genes (STING). The STING protein can be activated by cyclic dinucleotides (CDNs), which can be natural or synthetic. Injection of CDNs in mouse models of HNSCC resulted in robust antitumor immune responses, which were further enhanced by adding anti–PD-1 therapy.[50,51] Clinical trials of CDNs in combination with checkpoint inhibitors are currently underway.[51,52]

Inhibition of immunosuppressive cells

Some of the immune cells found within the tumor microenvironment are primarily immunosuppressive. These cells include myeloid-derived suppressor cells (MDSCs), regulatory T cells (Tregs), and M2 macrophages. Strategies under investigation for inhibiting MDSCs include specifically depleting them, preventing them from trafficking into the tumor, and impairing their function.[53–55] Treatments designed to deplete or inhibit Tregs or M2 macrophages have also been explored.[56,57]

Combination therapies

Based on the small proportion of patients with R/M disease who respond favorably to immune checkpoint blockade, more recent clinical trials have attempted to increase response rates by combining multiple forms of immunotherapy, or by combining immunotherapy with standard therapies. It has also been recognized that immunotherapy could be used strategically to increase response and survival rates in patients with high-risk, previously untreated, HPV-negative HNSCC, or to deescalate therapy for patients with HPV-related HNSCC.

Combinations of immunotherapy. Immunotherapeutic combinations may consist of multiple coinhibitory checkpoint inhibitors, or a coinhibitory checkpoint inhibitor in combination with a costimulatory agonist. Although combinations of anti–PD-1/PD-L1 and anti–CTLA-4 therapies have been useful for melanoma, similar combinations have shown disappointing results in HNSCC.[15,58] Combinations of the IDO1 inhibitor epacadostat with anti–PD-1 antibodies have shown some responses and favorable toxicity profiles.[59,60] As detailed earlier, STING and TLR agonists have also been used in combination with PD-1 inhibitors.

Immunotherapy combined with standard therapy. Standard therapies, such as chemotherapy and radiation, may enhance the antitumor immune response in HNSCC and other cancers. When radiation or chemotherapy are used, dying cancer cells release antigens and DAMPs, which can then be detected by immune cells. As a result, the tumor itself serves as an in situ vaccine. Preclinical studies in mouse tumor models have shown that radiation and platinum-based chemotherapy can enhance immunogenic cell death, antigen processing/presentation, and adaptive immunity.[61–69] Radiation used at one tumor site can result in responses at distant tumor sites outside the radiation field, a phenomenon known as the abscopal effect. The abscopal effect is mediated in large part by CD8+ T cells and may be enhanced by combining radiation with immune checkpoint blockade.[70–73] Multiple clinical trials have used reirradiation in combination with checkpoint inhibitors in the recurrent/metastatic setting for HNSCC and other solid tumors. For patients with previously untreated, locally advanced disease who are not eligible to receive cisplatin, anti–PD-1/PD-L1 antibodies alone or in combination with anti–CTLA-4 therapy have been used with radiation, so far with favorable results.[74–76] Larger studies are needed to compare the efficacy of these regimens with standard radiation plus cisplatin or cetuximab.

Platinum chemotherapy has been used successfully in combination with PD-1 inhibitors, first in lung cancer, and more recently in HNSCC. Initially, PD-1 inhibitors were only FDA approved for patients who had failed treatment with platinum-based chemotherapy. In the KEYNOTE-048 trial, patients were randomized to 1 of 3 arms: (1) the EXTREME regimen (cisplatin, fluorouracil and cetuximab), (2) first-line pembrolizumab (anti–PD-1), or (3) pembrolizumab (instead of cetuximab) in combination with cytotoxic chemotherapy (platinum/fluorouracil). At the second interim analysis, improved overall survival was noted with pembrolizumab alone in patients with PD-L1–positive tumors (CPS $\geq$ 1), leading to FDA approval of pembrolizumab as first-line therapy in 2019. The final analysis showed response and survival rates that were better with pembrolizumab/chemotherapy versus cetuximab/chemotherapy (EXTREME), regardless of PD-L1 status.[77] Based on these results from KEYNOTE-048, the current standard of care for recurrent/metastatic HNSCC is pembrolizumab alone for patients with PD-L1–positive tumors (CPS $\geq$ 1) and pembrolizumab plus chemotherapy for tumors with low expression of PD-L1 (CPS < 1). According to this scoring system, most patients with R/M disease are eligible for first-line pembrolizumab, which is far better tolerated than cytotoxic chemotherapy.

Because PD-1 inhibitors pair well with radiation and with chemotherapy, a logical next step was to combine all three modalities as a potential way of improving survival rates in patients with high-risk disease. In one study, pembrolizumab was added to radiation and low-dose, weekly cisplatin. This regimen was well tolerated and feasible, with most patients receiving the intended total doses of radiation and cisplatin.[78] In RTOG 3504, the addition of nivolumab to radiation with or without cisplatin or cetuximab was also safe and feasible.[79] However, these studies have not provided much information about efficacy of these regimens compared with chemoradiation alone. In the phase III JAVELIN head and neck 100 study, the addition of avelumab (anti–PD-L1) during and after cisplatin chemoradiation showed no added benefit versus chemoradiation plus placebo.[80] Although the reasons for this negative result are under debate, preclinical studies suggest that radiation is more likely to enhance the antitumor immune response when given in fewer, larger doses.[72,73] In contrast, cisplatin enhances the immune response when used in small weekly doses.[65] Thus, the standard radiation fractionation (2 Gy daily for 35 fractions) and high-dose cisplatin that are typically used for HNSCC may not be the optimal regimen for pairing with anti–PD-1/PD-L1 therapy.

Another way to enhance response rates to PD-1 checkpoint inhibitors is to administer them before surgery (neoadjuvant). Preclinical studies suggest neoadjuvant is more effective than adjuvant administration, likely because of the presence of anti–PD-1–responsive tumor infiltrating lymphocytes.[81] Response rates to neoadjuvant immune checkpoint blockade seem to be much higher than those seen in patients with R/M HNSCC.[82,83] Phase II studies using pembrolizumab or nivolumab in the neoadjuvant setting for high-risk HNSCC have shown acceptable toxicity, and delay in the timing of surgery has been uncommon. Pathologic responses were seen in more than 40% of surgical specimens, and some complete pathologic responses have been noted.[82–84] A phase III study of neoadjuvant and adjuvant pembrolizumab for patients with high-risk, surgically resectable HNSCC (KEYNOTE-689) is currently enrolling at multiple centers.[85]

CLINICS CARE POINTS

- Head and neck cancers may respond well to immunotherapy based on a high number of mutations and, in the case of HPV-positive disease, the presence of viral antigens.
- Patients with recurrent or metastatic HNSCC can be treated with PD-1 checkpoint inhibitors, which have fewer side effects than cytotoxic chemotherapy.
- Patients with recurrent/metastatic head and neck cancers that do not express PD-L1 are treated with PD-1 inhibition in addition to cytotoxic chemotherapy.
- In addition to immune checkpoint inhibitors, several other immunotherapeutic strategies are under rigorous investigation in numerous clinical trials.
- PD-1 immune checkpoint inhibitors can enhance the activity of chemotherapy and radiation, but the combination of all three modalities has been disappointing thus far.
- The use of neoadjuvant (presurgical) PD-1 immune checkpoint inhibitors seems to be a promising strategy for high-risk HNSCC.

DISCLOSURE

N.C. Schmitt: advisory board for Checkpoint Surgical; book royalties from Plural Publishing.

REFERENCES

1. Marincola FM, Lotze MT. Basic sciences - cracking the code of cancer immune responsiveness and evolution of cancer biology. In: Butterfield LH, Kaufman HL, Marincola FM, editors. Cancer immunotherapy principles and practice. New York: New York Demos Medical; 2017. p. 21–9.
2. Vermorken JB, Psyrri A, Mesia R, et al. Impact of tumor HPV status on outcome in patients with recurrent and/or metastatic squamous cell carcinoma of the head and neck receiving chemotherapy with or without cetuximab: retrospective analysis of the phase III EXTREME trial. Ann Oncol 2014;25(4):801–7.
3. Bonner JA, Harari PM, Giralt J, et al. Radiotherapy plus cetuximab for squamous-cell carcinoma of the head and neck. N Engl J Med 2006;354(6):567–78.
4. Ferris RL, Jaffee EM, Ferrone S. Tumor antigen-targeted, monoclonal antibody-based immunotherapy: clinical response, cellular immunity, and immunoescape. J Clin Oncol 2010;28(28):4390–9.
5. Lopez-Albaitero A, Lee SC, Morgan S, et al. Role of polymorphic Fc gamma receptor IIIa and EGFR expression level in cetuximab mediated, NK cell dependent in vitro cytotoxicity of head and neck squamous cell carcinoma cells. Cancer Immunol Immunother 2009;58(11):1853–64.
6. Srivastava RM, Lee SC, Andrade Filho PA, et al. Cetuximab-activated natural killer and dendritic cells collaborate to trigger tumor antigen-specific T-cell immunity in head and neck cancer patients. Clin Cancer Res 2013;19(7):1858–72.
7. Ferris RL, Kim S, Trivedi S, et al. Correlation of anti-tumor adaptive immunity with clinical response in phase II "window" trial of neoadjuvant cetuximab in patients

with resectable stage III-IV head and neck squamous cell carcinoma (HNSCC). J Clin Oncol 2016;34(suppl) [abstract: 6060].
8. Vermorken JB, Mesia R, Rivera F, et al. Platinum-based chemotherapy plus cetuximab in head and neck cancer. N Engl J Med 2008;359(11):1116–27.
9. Chow LQM, Haddad R, Gupta S, et al. Antitumor Activity of Pembrolizumab in Biomarker-Unselected Patients With Recurrent and/or Metastatic Head and Neck Squamous Cell Carcinoma: Results From the Phase Ib KEYNOTE-012 Expansion Cohort. J Clin Oncol 2016;34(32):3838–45.
10. Mehra R, Seiwert TY, Gupta S, et al. Efficacy and safety of pembrolizumab in recurrent/metastatic head and neck squamous cell carcinoma: pooled analyses after long-term follow-up in KEYNOTE-012. Br J Cancer 2018;119(2):153–9.
11. Ferris RL, Blumenschein G Jr, Fayette J, et al. Nivolumab for Recurrent Squamous-Cell Carcinoma of the Head and Neck. N Engl J Med 2016;375(19): 1856–67.
12. Cohen EEW, Soulières D, Le Tourneau C, et al. Pembrolizumab versus methotrexate, docetaxel, or cetuximab for recurrent or metastatic head-and-neck squamous cell carcinoma (KEYNOTE-040): a randomised, open-label, phase 3 study. Lancet 2019;393(10167):156–67.
13. Segal NH, Ou SI, Balmanoukian A, et al. Safety and efficacy of durvalumab in patients with head and neck squamous cell carcinoma: results from a phase I/II expansion cohort. Eur J Cancer 2019;109:154–61.
14. Ferris RL, Blumenschein G Jr, Fayette J, et al. Nivolumab vs investigator's choice in recurrent or metastatic squamous cell carcinoma of the head and neck: 2-year long-term survival update of CheckMate 141 with analyses by tumor PD-L1 expression. Oral Oncol 2018;81:45–51.
15. Zandberg DP, Algazi AP, Jimeno A, et al. Durvalumab for recurrent or metastatic head and neck squamous cell carcinoma: Results from a single-arm, phase II study in patients with >/=25% tumour cell PD-L1 expression who have progressed on platinum-based chemotherapy. Eur J Cancer 2019;107:142–52.
16. Wang J, Sun H, Zeng Q, et al. HPV-positive status associated with inflamed immune microenvironment and improved response to anti-PD-1 therapy in head and neck squamous cell carcinoma. Sci Rep 2019;9(1):13404.
17. Kansy BA, Concha-Benavente F, Srivastava RM, et al. PD-1 Status in CD8(+) T Cells Associates with Survival and Anti-PD-1 Therapeutic Outcomes in Head and Neck Cancer. Cancer Res 2017;77(22):6353–64.
18. Larkin J, Chiarion-Sileni V, Gonzalez R, et al. Five-year survival with combined nivolumab and ipilimumab in advanced melanoma. N Engl J Med 2019;381(16): 1535–46.
19. Siu LL, Even C, Mesia R, et al. Safety and efficacy of durvalumab with or without tremelimumab in patients with PD-L1-low/negative recurrent or metastatic HNSCC: The Phase 2 CONDOR Randomized Clinical Trial. JAMA Oncol 2019; 5(2):195–203.
20. Gameiro SF, Ghasemi F, Barrett JW, et al. Treatment-naive HPV+ head and neck cancers display a T-cell-inflamed phenotype distinct from their HPV- counterparts that has implications for immunotherapy. Oncoimmunology 2018;7(10): e1498439.
21. Wirth L, Burtness B, Mehra R, et al. IDO1 as a mechanism of adaptive immune resistance to anti-PD-1 monotherapy in HNSCC. J Clin Oncol 2017;35(suppl): 2017 [abstract: 6053].

22. Wu L, Mao L, Liu JF, et al. Blockade of TIGIT/CD155 signaling reverses T-cell exhaustion and enhances antitumor capability in head and neck squamous cell carcinoma. Cancer Immunol Res 2019;7(10):1700–13.
23. Oweida A, Hararah MK, Phan A, et al. Resistance to radiotherapy and PD-L1 blockade is mediated by TIM-3 upregulation and regulatory T-cell infiltration. Clin Cancer Res 2018;24(21):5368–80.
24. Pfannenstiel LW, Diaz-Montero CM, Tian YF, et al. Immune-Checkpoint Blockade Opposes CD8(+) T-cell Suppression in Human and Murine Cancer. Cancer Immunol Res 2019;7(3):510–25.
25. Liu Z, McMichael EL, Shayan G, et al. Novel effector phenotype of tim-3(+) regulatory t cells leads to enhanced suppressive function in head and neck cancer patients. Clin Cancer Res 2018;24(18):4529–38.
26. Woo SR, Turnis ME, Goldberg MV, et al. Immune inhibitory molecules LAG-3 and PD-1 synergistically regulate T-cell function to promote tumoral immune escape. Cancer Res 2012;72(4):917–27.
27. Bell RB, Leidner RS, Crittenden MR, et al. OX40 signaling in head and neck squamous cell carcinoma: Overcoming immunosuppression in the tumor microenvironment. Oral Oncol 2016;52:1–10.
28. Baruah P, Lee M, Odutoye T, et al. Decreased levels of alternative co-stimulatory receptors OX40 and 4-1BB characterise T cells from head and neck cancer patients. Immunobiology 2012;217(7):669–75.
29. Lucido CT, Vermeer PD, Wieking BG, et al. CD137 enhancement of HPV positive head and neck squamous cell carcinoma tumor clearance. Vaccines (Basel) 2014;2(4):841–53.
30. Voskens CJ, Sewell D, Hertzano R, et al. Induction of MAGE-A3 and HPV-16 immunity by Trojan vaccines in patients with head and neck carcinoma. Head Neck 2012;34(12):1734–46.
31. Gildener-Leapman N, Lee J, Ferris RL. Tailored immunotherapy for HPV positive head and neck squamous cell cancer. Oral Oncol 2014;50(9):780–4.
32. Reuschenbach M, Pauligk C, Karbach J, et al. A phase 1/2a study to test the safety and immunogenicity of a p16(INK4a) peptide vaccine in patients with advanced human papillomavirus-associated cancers. Cancer 2016;122(9): 1425–33.
33. Aggarwal C, Halmos B, Porosnicu M, et al. A phase 1b/2a, multi-center, open-label study to evaluate the safety and efficacy of combination treatment with MEDI0457 (INO-3112) and durvalumab (MEDI4736) in patients with recurrent/ metastatic human papilloma virus-associated head and neck squamous cell cancer. J Clin Oncol 2018;36(suppl):2018 [abstr: TPS6093].
34. Sacco JJ, Evans M, Harrington KJ, et al. Systemic listeriosis following vaccination with the attenuated Listeria monocytogenes therapeutic vaccine, ADXS11-001. Hum Vaccin Immunother 2016;12(4):1085–6.
35. Hennessy ML, Bommareddy PK, Boland G, et al. Oncolytic Immunotherapy. Surg Oncol Clin N Am 2019;28(3):419–30.
36. Ribas A, Dummer R, Puzanov I, et al. Oncolytic virotherapy promotes intratumoral T cell infiltration and improves anti-PD-1 immunotherapy. Cell 2018;174(4): 1031–2.
37. Harrington KJ, Hingorani M, Tanay MA, et al. Phase I/II study of oncolytic HSV GM-CSF in combination with radiotherapy and cisplatin in untreated stage III/IV squamous cell cancer of the head and neck. Clin Cancer Res 2010;16(15): 4005–15.

38. Mell LK, Brumund KT, Daniels GA, et al. Phase I trial of intravenous oncolytic vaccinia virus (GL-ONC1) with cisplatin and radiotherapy in patients with locoregionally advanced head and neck carcinoma. Clin Cancer Res 2017;23(19): 5696–702.
39. Stevanovic S, Draper LM, Langhan MM, et al. Complete regression of metastatic cervical cancer after treatment with human papillomavirus-targeted tumor-infiltrating T cells. J Clin Oncol 2015;33(14):1543–50.
40. Doran SL, Stevanovic S, Adhikary S, et al. T-cell receptor gene therapy for human papillomavirus-associated epithelial cancers: A first-in-human, phase I/II study. J Clin Oncol 2019;37(30):2759–69.
41. van Schalkwyk MC, Papa SE, Jeannon JP, et al. Design of a phase I clinical trial to evaluate intratumoral delivery of ErbB-targeted chimeric antigen receptor T-cells in locally advanced or recurrent head and neck cancer. Hum Gene Ther Clin Dev 2013;24(3):134–42.
42. Friedman J, Padget M, Lee J, et al. Direct and antibody-dependent cell-mediated cytotoxicity of head and neck squamous cell carcinoma cells by high-affinity natural killer cells. Oral Oncol 2019;90:38–44.
43. Jouhi L, Mohamed H, Makitie A, et al. Toll-like receptor 5 and 7 expression may impact prognosis of HPV-positive oropharyngeal squamous cell carcinoma patients. Cancer Immunol Immunother 2017;66(12):1619–29.
44. Stephenson RM, Lim CM, Matthews M, et al. TLR8 stimulation enhances cetuximab-mediated natural killer cell lysis of head and neck cancer cells and dendritic cell cross-priming of EGFR-specific CD8+ T cells. Cancer Immunol Immunother 2013;62(8):1347–57.
45. Dietsch GN, Lu H, Yang Y, et al. Coordinated Activation of Toll-Like Receptor8 (TLR8) and NLRP3 by the TLR8 Agonist, VTX-2337, Ignites Tumoricidal Natural Killer Cell Activity. PLoS One 2016;11(2):e0148764.
46. Sato-Kaneko F, Yao S, Ahmadi A, et al. Combination immunotherapy with TLR agonists and checkpoint inhibitors suppresses head and neck cancer. JCI Insight 2017;2(18):e93397.
47. Chow LQM, Morishima C, Eaton KD, et al. Phase Ib Trial of the Toll-like Receptor 8 Agonist, Motolimod (VTX-2337), Combined with Cetuximab in Patients with Recurrent or Metastatic SCCHN. Clin Cancer Res 2017;23(10):2442–50.
48. Ferris RL, Saba NF, Gitlitz BJ, et al. Effect of adding motolimod to standard combination chemotherapy and cetuximab treatment of patients with squamous cell carcinoma of the head and neck: the active8 randomized clinical trial. JAMA Oncol 2018;4(11):1583–8.
49. Cohen EE, Nabell L, Wong DJL, et al. Phase 1b/2, open label, multicenter study of intratumoral SD-101 in combination with pembrolizumab in anti-PD-1 treatment naïve patients with recurrent or metastatic head and neck squamous cell carcinoma (HNSCC). J Clin Oncol 2019;37(suppl):2019 [abstract: 6039].
50. Gadkaree SK, Fu J, Sen R, et al. Induction of tumor regression by intratumoral STING agonists combined with anti-programmed death-L1 blocking antibody in a preclinical squamous cell carcinoma model. Head Neck 2017;39(6):1086–94.
51. Moore E, Clavijo PE, Davis R, et al. Established T cell-inflamed tumors rejected after adaptive resistance was reversed by combination STING activation and PD-1 pathway blockade. Cancer Immunol Res 2016;4(12):1061–71.
52. Harrington KJ, Brody J, Ingham M, et al. Preliminary results of the first-in-human (FIH) study of MK-1454, an agonist of stimulator of interferon genes (STING), as monotherapy or in combination with pembrolizumab (pembro) in patients with advanced solid tumors or lymphomas. Ann Oncol 2018;29(suppl_8).

53. Clavijo PE, Moore EC, Chen J, et al. Resistance to CTLA-4 checkpoint inhibition reversed through selective elimination of granulocytic myeloid cells. Oncotarget 2017;8(34):55804–20.
54. Davis RJ, Moore EC, Clavijo PE, et al. Anti-PD-L1 Efficacy Can Be Enhanced by Inhibition of Myeloid-Derived Suppressor Cells with a Selective Inhibitor of PI3K-delta/gamma. Cancer Res 2017;77(10):2607–19.
55. Sun L, Clavijo PE, Robbins Y, et al. Inhibiting myeloid-derived suppressor cell trafficking enhances T cell immunotherapy. JCI Insight 2019;4(7):e126853.
56. Ye W, Schmitt NC, Ferris RL, et al. Improving responses to immunotherapy in head and neck squamous cell carcinoma. In: Kimple RJ, editor. Improving the therapeutic ration in head and neck cancer. San Diego (CA): Elsevier; 2020. p. 107–33.
57. Zhu Y, Knolhoff BL, Meyer MA, et al. CSF1/CSF1R blockade reprograms tumor-infiltrating macrophages and improves response to T-cell checkpoint immunotherapy in pancreatic cancer models. Cancer Res 2014;74(18):5057–69.
58. Ferris RL, Haddad R, Even C, et al. Durvalumab with or without tremelimumab in patients with recurrent or metastatic head and neck squamous cell carcinoma: EAGLE, a randomized, open-label phase III study. Ann Oncol 2020;31(7):942–50.
59. Daud A, Saleh MN, Hu J, et al. Epacadostat plus nivolumab for advanced melanoma: Updated phase 2 results of the ECHO-204 study. J Clin Oncol 2018; 36(suppl):2018 [abstract: 9511].
60. Hamid O, Bauer TM, Spira AI, et al. Epacadostat plus pembrolizumab in patients with SCCHN: Preliminary phase 1/2 results from ECHO-202/KEYNOTE-037. J Clin Oncol 2017;35(suppl):2017 [abstract: 6010].
61. de Biasi AR, Villena-Vargas J, Adusumilli PS. Cisplatin-induced antitumor immunomodulation: a review of preclinical and clinical evidence. Clin Cancer Res 2014;20(21):5384–91.
62. Dovedi SJ, Illidge TM. The antitumor immune response generated by fractionated radiation therapy may be limited by tumor cell adaptive resistance and can be circumvented by PD-L1 blockade. Oncoimmunology 2015;4(7):e1016709.
63. Hato SV, Khong A, de Vries IJ, et al. Molecular pathways: the immunogenic effects of platinum-based chemotherapeutics. Clin Cancer Res 2014;20(11):2831–7.
64. Spanos WC, Nowicki P, Lee DW, et al. Immune response during therapy with cisplatin or radiation for human papillomavirus-related head and neck cancer. Arch Otolaryngol Head Neck Surg 2009;135(11):1137–46.
65. Tran L, Allen CT, Xiao R, et al. Cisplatin alters antitumor immunity and synergizes with PD-1/PD-L1 inhibition in head and neck squamous cell carcinoma. Cancer Immunol Res 2017;5(12):1141–51.
66. Park SJ, Ye W, Xiao R, et al. Cisplatin and oxaliplatin induce similar immunogenic changes in preclinical models of head and neck cancer. Oral Oncol 2019;95:127–35.
67. Bezu L, Gomes-de-Silva LC, Dewitte H, et al. Combinatorial strategies for the induction of immunogenic cell death. Front Immunol 2015;6:187.
68. Kepp O, Galluzzi L, Martins I, et al. Molecular determinants of immunogenic cell death elicited by anticancer chemotherapy. Cancer Metastasis Rev 2011; 30(1):61–9.
69. Martins I, Kepp O, Schlemmer F, et al. Restoration of the immunogenicity of cisplatin-induced cancer cell death by endoplasmic reticulum stress. Oncogene 2011;30(10):1147–58.
70. Ferris RL. Immunology and immunotherapy of head and neck cancer. J Clin Oncol 2015;33(29):3293–304.
71. Schoppy DW, Sunwoo JB. Immunotherapy for head and neck squamous cell carcinoma. Hematol Oncol Clin North Am 2015;29(6):1033–43.

72. Morisada M, Clavijo PE, Moore E, et al. PD-1 blockade reverses adaptive immune resistance induced by high-dose hypofractionated but not low-dose daily fractionated radiation. Oncoimmunology 2018;7(3):e1395996.
73. Buchwald ZS, Wynne J, Nasti TH, et al. Radiation, immune checkpoint blockade and the abscopal effect: a critical review on timing, dose and fractionation. Front Oncol 2018;8:612.
74. Johnson JM, Ad VB, Lorber E, et al. Safety of nivolumab and ipilimumab in combination with radiotherapy in patients with locally advanced squamous cell carcinoma of the head and neck (LA SCCHN). J Clin Oncol 2019;37(suppl):2019 [abstract: 6070].
75. Mell LK, Torres-Saavedra PA, Wong SJ, et al. Safety of radiotherapy with concurrent and adjuvant MEDI4736 (durvalumab) in patients with locoregionally advanced head and neck cancer with a contraindication to cisplatin: NRG-HN004. J Clin Oncol 2019;37(suppl):2019 [abstract: 6065].
76. Weiss J, Sheth S, Deal AM, et al. Concurrent definitive immunoradiotherapy for patients with stage III-IV head and neck cancer and cisplatin contraindication. Clin Cancer Res 2020;26(16):4260–7.
77. Burtness B, Harrington KJ, Greil R, et al. Pembrolizumab alone or with chemotherapy versus cetuximab with chemotherapy for recurrent or metastatic squamous cell carcinoma of the head and neck (KEYNOTE-048): a randomised, open-label, phase 3 study. Lancet 2019;394(10212):1915–28.
78. Powell SF, Gold KA, Gitau MM, et al. Safety and efficacy of pembrolizumab with chemoradiotherapy in locally advanced head and neck squamous cell carcinoma: a phase IB study. J Clin Oncol 2020;38:2427–37.
79. Gillison ML, Ferris RL, Harris J, et al. Safety and disease control achieved with the addition of nivolumab (Nivo) to chemoradiotherapy (CRT) for intermediate (IR) and high-risk (HR) local-regionally advanced head and neck squamous cell carcinoma (HNSCC): RTOG Foundation 3504. J Clin Oncol 2019;37(suppl):2019 [abstract: 6073].
80. Cohen EE, Ferris RL, Psyrri A, et al. Primary results of the phase III JAVELIN head & neck 100 trial: Avelumab plus chemoradiotherapy (CRT) followed by avelumab maintenance vs CRT in patients with locally advanced squamous cell carcinoma of the head and neck (LA SCCHN). Ann Oncol 2020;31:S658.
81. Friedman J, Moore E, Zolkind P, et al. Neoadjuvant PD-1 immune checkpoint blockade reverses functional immunodominance among tumor-antigen specific T cells. Clin Cancer Res 2019. https://doi.org/10.1158/1078-0432.
82. Uppaluri R, Campbell KM, Egloff AM, et al. Neoadjuvant and adjuvant pembrolizumab in resectable locally advanced, human papillomavirus-unrelated head and neck cancer: a multicenter, phase II trial. Clin Cancer Res 2020;26(19): 5140–52.
83. Xiong Y, Neskey DM, Horton JD, et al. Immunological effects of nivolumab immunotherapy in patients with oral cavity squamous cell carcinoma. BMC Cancer 2020;20(1):229.
84. Wise-Draper TM, Old MO, Worden F, et al. Phase II multi-site investigation of neoadjuvant pembrolizumab and adjuvant concurrent radiation and pembrolizumab with or without cisplatin in resected head and neck squamous cell carcinoma. J Clin Oncol 2018;36(suppl):2018 [abstract: 6017].
85. Uppaluri R, Lee NY, Westra W, et al. KEYNOTE-689: Phase 3 study of adjuvant and neoadjuvant pembrolizumab combined with standard of care (SOC) in patients with resectable, locally advanced head and neck squamous cell carcinoma. J Clin Oncol 2019;37(suppl) [abstract: TPS6090].

Epidermal Growth Factor Receptor-Targeted Therapy for Head and Neck Cancer

Sumita Trivedi, MD[a], Robert L. Ferris, MD, PhD[b,c,d,*]

KEYWORDS

- Epidermal growth factor receptor • Monoclonal antibody • Cetuximab
- Tyrosine kinase inhibitor

KEY POINTS

- The epidermal growth factor receptor (EGFR) is overexpressed in most head and neck cancers and associated with poor survival outcomes.
- The 2 main classes of drugs that target EGFR include anti-EGFR monoclonal antibodies and small molecule tyrosine kinase inhibitors.
- Cetuximab, an anti-EGFR monoclonal antibody, is approved for use in local/regional advanced and recurrent or metastatic head and neck cancer.
- Other anti-EGFR monoclonal antibodies and tyrosine kinase inhibitors have been evaluated for use in head and neck cancers

The epidermal growth factor receptor (EGFR) is a member of the ErbB receptor family, which regulates several pathways that promote tumorigenesis. Membrane-bound EGFR complexed with its natural ligands, EGF, or transforming growth factor alpha (TGF-α), results in homodimerization with other EGFR molecules or heterodimerization with other ErbB family members. This subsequently activates intracellular tyrosine kinase signaling pathways leading to proliferation, angiogenesis, antiapoptosis, and metastasis in malignant cells.[1,2] EGFR overexpression occurs in 80% to 90% of head and neck squamous cell carcinomas (HNSCC) and is associated with poor survival outcomes.[3,4] EGFR targeting represents an appealing therapeutic strategy, and several studies have evaluated the 2 main classes of drugs targeting EGFR, monoclonal antibodies (mAb) and small molecule tyrosine kinase inhibitors (TKIs) in HNSCC.

[a] Division of Hematology/Oncology, Department of Medicine, University of Pennsylvania, Philadelphia, PA, USA; [b] Department of Otolaryngology, University of Pittsburgh, Pittsburgh, PA, USA; [c] Department of Immunology, University of Pittsburgh, Pittsburgh, PA, USA; [d] UPMC Hillman Cancer Center, Pittsburgh, USA

* Corresponding author. Hillman Cancer Center, 5115 Centre Avenue, Suite 500, Pittsburgh, PA 15213-1863.

E-mail address: ferrrl@upmc.edu

Otolaryngol Clin N Am 54 (2021) 743–749
https://doi.org/10.1016/j.otc.2021.04.005

Cetuximab is a mouse-human chimeric immunoglobulin G1 (IgG1) anti-EGFR mAb that acts to inhibit ligand binding to the EGFR and enhances the activity of chemotherapeutic agents.[5,6] It additionally functions to enhance antitumor immune activity by stimulating antibody-dependent cell-mediated cytotoxicity (ADCC) and T cell priming.[7] IgG1 isotype mAbs have been shown to augment immune cell targeting and killing of antibody-coated cells in the presence of NK cells.[8] The process of ADCC is initiated when the Fc region of cetuximab binds to the activating CD16 Fc receptor on the NK cell. Once activated, NK cells can directly kill tumors cells, releasing tumor antigens that can be presented by dendritic cells to prime T cells for additional tumor killing.[9] Activated NK cells additionally release cytokines to facilitate cross-talk with dendritic cells and other immune cells that draw cytotoxic T cells to the tumor microenvironment via chemoattraction.[10,11]

In 2006, concurrent cetuximab-sensitized radiation became an approved standard therapy for patients with local/regional advanced HNSCC based on data that demonstrated improved locoregional control and overall survival (OS) compared with radiation alone.[12] Bonner and colleagues[13] randomized 424 patients with locally advanced HNSCC to receive definitive radiation with or without cetuximab. Locoregional control and median OS were significantly improved in patients who received the concurrent cetuximab with radiation compared with radiation alone (49 months vs 29.3 months, *P*=.03). At 5 years, OS in patients treated with cetuximab and radiation was 45.6% compared with 36.4% in those treated with radiation alone (hazard ratio [HR] 0.73, 95% confidence interval [CI], 0.56–0.95, *P*=.018).[14]

Interest in deintensification treatment strategies for human papillomavirus (HPV)-positive HNSCC resulted in several trials comparing cetuximab with cisplatin as a radiation sensitizer. Results of these trials show decreased survival with concurrent cetuximab-sensitized radiation compared to cisplatin-sensitized radiation. RTOG 1016 was a noninferiority trial of 849 patients with locally advanced HPV-positive oropharyngeal cancer who were randomized to receive radiation with either cetuximab or cisplatin. At 4.5-year median follow-up, the cetuximab arm did not meet criteria for noninferiority, with a 5-year OS of 77.9% compared with 84.6% for the cisplatin arm.[15] In the phase III De-ESCALaTE trial, cetuximab or cisplatin in combination with radiation was compared in 334 patients with locally advanced HPV-positive oropharyngeal cancer. Two-year OS was significantly improved in patients who received cisplatin (97.5%) compared with cetuximab (89.4%).[16] Concurrent cetuximab radiation remains the treatment of choice for patients with HPV-negative locally advanced HNSCC who are ineligible for cisplatin.

In 2011, cetuximab was approved for recurrent or metastatic HNSCC in combination with platinum-based chemotherapy and fluorouracil based on results of the phase III EXTREME trial.[17] Patents were assigned to receive either cisplatin/5-FU or carboplatin/5-FU either alone or with cetuximab. The addition of cetuximab improved median survival compared with the standard chemotherapy doublet of platinum/5-FU (10.1 vs 7.4 months, *P*=.04).

Based on the findings with cetuximab, panitumumab, a fully humanized immunoglobulin G2 (IgG2) anti-EGFR mAb was evaluated in several trials in HNSCC. CONCERT-1, a phase II trial randomized 150 patients with unresected, locally advanced HNSCC to either chemoradiotherapy or panitumumab with chemoradiotherapy and found that the addition of panitumumab did not confer clinical benefit. Locoregional control at 2 years in the chemoradiotherapy group was 68% compared with 61% in the panitumumab with chemoradiotherapy group.[18] CONCERT-2 compared panitumumab and radiation with cisplatin and radiation in patients with locally advanced HNSCC. Locoregional control at 2 years was 61% with cisplatin and radiation compared to 51% with panitumumab and radiation.[19] In patients with recurrent or metastatic HNSCC, the addition of panitumumab to cisplatin and fluorouracil was not found to improve overall survival in the phase III SPECTRUM trial. Median OS was 11.1 months (95% CI 9.8–12.2) in the panitumumab group and 9.0 months (8.1–11.2 months) in the cisplatin/5-FU group (HR 0.873, 95% CI 0.729–1.046; *P*=0.1403). Median progression-free survival was 5.8 months (95% CI 5.6–6.6) in the panitumumab group and 4.6 months (4.1–5.4) in the cisplatin/5-FU group (HR 0.780, 95% CI 0.659–0.922; *P*=0.0036).[20] This differing efficacy of cetuximab and panitumumab in patients may be a result of the mAb-dependent immune mechanisms associated with cetuximab that are not induced by panitumumab. The IgG2 isotype mAb does not trigger NK cell-mediated ADCC.[21,22]

TKIs act within the intracellular tyrosine kinase domain of EGFR, competing with ATP to eliminate EGFR downstream signaling. They are short-acting oral agents that have been approved for use in nonsmall cell lung cancer. TKIs have been evaluated in locally advanced HNSCC and have not demonstrated improvement in either progression-free survival or response rates. Erlotinib combined with definitive cisplatin and radiation was compared with definitive cisplatin and radiation in a phase II trial of 205 patients with locally advanced HNSCC. A complete response rate of 40% was found in patients who received cisplatin and radiation and 52% in those who received erlotinib with cisplatin and radiation (*P*=.08); no difference in progression-free survival was noted (HR, 0.9 *P*=.71).[23] In the adjuvant setting, afatinib was compared with placebo in a phase III trial of 617 patients following definitive chemoradiation or chemo radiation and surgery for locally advanced HNSCC. Median disease-free survival was 43.4 months (95% CI, 37.4 months to not estimable) in the afatinib group and not estimable (95% CI, 40.1 months to not estimable) in the placebo group (HR 1.13 95% CI, 0.81–1.57, *P*=.48).[24] Several TKIs including gefitinib, erlotinib, lapatinib and tivantinib have been evaluated in the recurrent and metastatic setting without demonstrable effect.[25–27] Large phase III trials comparing gefitinib and afatinib alone and in combination with docetaxel to standard chemotherapy were without significant improvement in OS.[28,29] The lack of efficacy of TKIs in HNSCC is partially explained by the lack of activating EGFR mutations seen in HNSCC compared with nonsmall cell lung cancer.[30,31]

Despite promising preclinical studies, only a small subset of patients derives clinical benefit from EGFR inhibition. Furthermore, patients who initially respond to EGFR inhibition may subsequently become refractory because of the development of acquired inhibitor resistance. Upregulation of HER3 signaling has been elucidated as a mechanism that underlies acquired resistance to cetuximab and gefitinib in HNSCC.[32–34] Phosphorylated HER3 activates downstream PI3K/AKT signaling and can form heterodimers with HER2 to further potentiate this effect. The combination of cetuximab with HER2 blockade may be a strategy to overcome cetuximab resistance.[35] Compensatory activation of the MET oncogene is another key mechanism that contributes to acquired resistance to cetuximab.[36] MET activates many of the same downstream signaling pathways as EGFR including PI3K/AKT and ERK1/2 and promotes tumor growth.[37] Ligand-independent MET activation has also been demonstrated in erlotinib and gefitinib-resistant HNSCC.[38,39] Blocking MET could be an important strategy to overcome resistance to EGFR-inhibition.[40] Other resistance mechanisms include loss of p53, induction of epithelial to mesenchymal transition, and alternate pathways to activate downstream signals such as RAS and PIK3CA mutations.[41–43]

EGFR remains an important therapeutic target in HNSCC because of overexpression in this disease and functions as an integral point for converging signaling pathways. Despite studies of multiple anti-EGFR mAbs and TKIs, only cetuximab has been US Food and Drug Administration (FDA) approved as a targeted agent for HNSCC. Acquired resistance mechanisms add complexity to the treatment paradigm, and combination therapies may be necessary to overcome these. Cetuximab mediates tumor cell apoptosis through direct EGFR inhibition combined with mAb-dependent immune activation. The immune effects of cetuximab appear to be integral to its efficacy in HNSCC and underline the importance of harnessing the immune system for successful therapy in this disease. As strategies for immunotherapy are optimized in HNSCC, the combination of cetuximab with immune checkpoint inhibitors could combine inhibition of tumorigenic pathways with upregulation of antitumor immune responses.

CLINICS CARE POINTS

- EGFR overexpression in HNSCC is associated with poor survival outcomes.
- Concurrent cetuximab with radiation remains the treatment of choice for patients with HPV-negative, local or regionally advanced HNSCC who are ineligible for cisplatin.
- In HPV-positive HNSCC, concurrent cetuximab with radiation demonstrates decreased overall survival compared to concurrent cisplatin with radiation.
- TKIs do not demonstrate significant efficacy in HNSCC, due in part to the lack of activating EGFR mutations in this disease.
- Combining therapeutic agents may be 1 strategy to reduce acquired resistance mechanisms to EGFR targeted therapy and improve outcomes.

DISCLOSURE

R.L. Ferris: Aduro Biotech, Inc: Consulting. Astra-Zeneca/MedImmune: Clinical Trial, Research Funding. Bristol-Myers Squibb: Advisory Board, Clinical Trial, Research Funding. EMD Serono: Advisory Board. MacroGenics, Inc: Advisory Board. Merck: Advisory Board, Clinical Trial. Novasenta: Consulting, Stock, Research Funding. Numab Therapeutics AG: Advisory Board. Pfizer: Advisory Board. Sanofi: Consultant. Tesaro: Research Funding. Zymeworks, Inc: Consultant.

REFERENCE

1. Kalyankrishna S, Grandis JR. Epidermal growth factor receptor biology in head and neck cancer. J Clin Oncol 2006;24(17):2666–72.
2. Roskoski R Jr. The ErbB/HER receptor protein-tyrosine kinases and cancer. Biochem Biophys Res Commun 2004;319(1):1–11.
3. Rubin Grandis J, Melhem MF, Gooding WE, et al. Levels of TGF-alpha and EGFR protein in head and neck squamous cell carcinoma and patient survival. J Natl Cancer Inst 1998;90(11):824–32.
4. Zhu X, Zhang F, Zhang W, et al. Prognostic role of epidermal growth factor receptor in head and neck cancer: a meta-analysis. J Surg Oncol 2013;108(6):387–97.
5. Li S, Schmitz KR, Jeffrey PD, et al. Structural basis for inhibition of the epidermal growth factor receptor by cetuximab. Cancer Cell 2005;7(4):301–11.
6. Fan Z, Baselga J, Masui H, et al. Antitumor effect of anti-epidermal growth factor receptor monoclonal antibodies plus cis-diamminedichloroplatinum on well established A431 cell xenografts. Cancer Res 1993;53(19):4637–42.

7. Chow LQM, Morishima C, Eaton KD, et al. Phase Ib trial of the toll-like receptor 8 agonist, motolimod (VTX-2337), combined with cetuximab in patients with recurrent or metastatic SCCHN. Clin Cancer Res 2017;23(10):2442–50.
8. Kimura H, Sakai K, Arao T, et al. Antibody-dependent cellular cytotoxicity of cetuximab against tumor cells with wild-type or mutant epidermal growth factor receptor. Cancer Sci 2007;98(8):1275–80.
9. Kroemer G, Galluzzi L, Kepp O, et al. Immunogenic cell death in cancer therapy. Annu Rev Immunol 2013;31:51–72.
10. Pozzi C, Cuomo A, Spadoni I, et al. The EGFR-specific antibody cetuximab combined with chemotherapy triggers immunogenic cell death. Nat Med 2016;22(6): 624–31.
11. Ferris RL, Lenz HJ, Trotta AM, et al. Rationale for combination of therapeutic antibodies targeting tumor cells and immune checkpoint receptors: Harnessing innate and adaptive immunity through IgG1 isotype immune effector stimulation. Cancer Treat Rev 2018;63:48–60.
12. Massarelli E, William W, Johnson F, et al. Combining immune checkpoint blockade and tumor-specific vaccine for patients with incurable human papillomavirus 16-related cancer: a phase 2 clinical trial. JAMA Oncol 2019;5(1):67–73.
13. Bonner JA, Harari PM, Giralt J, et al. Radiotherapy plus cetuximab for squamous-cell carcinoma of the head and neck. N Engl J Med 2006;354(6):567–78.
14. Bonner JA, Harari PM, Giralt J, et al. Radiotherapy plus cetuximab for locoregionally advanced head and neck cancer: 5-year survival data from a phase 3 randomised trial, and relation between cetuximab-induced rash and survival. Lancet Oncol 2010;11(1):21–8.
15. Gillison ML, Trotti AM, Harris J, et al. Radiotherapy plus cetuximab or cisplatin in human papillomavirus-positive oropharyngeal cancer (NRG Oncology RTOG 1016): a randomised, multicentre, non-inferiority trial. Lancet 2019;393(10166): 40–50.
16. Mehanna H, Robinson M, Hartley A, et al. Radiotherapy plus cisplatin or cetuximab in low-risk human papillomavirus-positive oropharyngeal cancer (De-ESCALaTE HPV): an open-label randomised controlled phase 3 trial. Lancet 2019; 393(10166):51–60.
17. Vermorken JB, Mesia R, Rivera F, et al. Platinum-based chemotherapy plus cetuximab in head and neck cancer. N Engl J Med 2008;359(11):1116–27.
18. Mesia R, Henke M, Fortin A, et al. Chemoradiotherapy with or without panitumumab in patients with unresected, locally advanced squamous-cell carcinoma of the head and neck (CONCERT-1): a randomised, controlled, open-label phase 2 trial. Lancet Oncol 2015;16(2):208–20.
19. Giralt J, Trigo J, Nuyts S, et al. Panitumumab plus radiotherapy versus chemoradiotherapy in patients with unresected, locally advanced squamous-cell carcinoma of the head and neck (CONCERT-2): a randomised, controlled, open-label phase 2 trial. Lancet Oncol 2015;16(2):221–32.
20. Vermorken JB, Stohlmacher-Williams J, Davidenko I, et al. Cisplatin and fluorouracil with or without panitumumab in patients with recurrent or metastatic squamous-cell carcinoma of the head and neck (SPECTRUM): an open-label phase 3 randomised trial. Lancet Oncol 2013;14(8):697–710.
21. Trivedi S, Srivastava RM, Concha-Benavente F, et al. Anti-EGFR targeted monoclonal antibody isotype influences antitumor cellular immunity in head and neck cancer patients. Clin Cancer Res 2016;22(21):5229–37.
22. Argiris A. EGFR inhibition for recurrent or metastatic HNSCC. Lancet Oncol 2015; 16(5):488–9.

23. Martins RG, Parvathaneni U, Bauman JE, et al. Cisplatin and radiotherapy with or without erlotinib in locally advanced squamous cell carcinoma of the head and neck: a randomized phase II trial. J Clin Oncol 2013;31(11):1415–21.
24. Burtness B, Haddad R, Dinis J, et al. Afatinib vs placebo as adjuvant therapy after chemoradiotherapy in squamous cell carcinoma of the head and neck: a randomized clinical trial. JAMA Oncol 2019;5(8):1170–80.
25. Soulieres D, Senzer NN, Vokes EE, et al. Multicenter phase II study of erlotinib, an oral epidermal growth factor receptor tyrosine kinase inhibitor, in patients with recurrent or metastatic squamous cell cancer of the head and neck. J Clin Oncol 2004;22(1):77–85.
26. Kochanny SE, Worden FP, Adkins DR, et al. A randomized phase 2 network trial of tivantinib plus cetuximab versus cetuximab in patients with recurrent/metastatic head and neck squamous cell carcinoma. Cancer 2020;126(10):2146–52.
27. Kirby AM, A'Hern RP, D'Ambrosio C, et al. Gefitinib (ZD1839, Iressa) as palliative treatment in recurrent or metastatic head and neck cancer. Br J Cancer 2006; 94(5):631–6.
28. Stewart JS, Cohen EE, Licitra L, et al. Phase III study of gefitinib compared with intravenous methotrexate for recurrent squamous cell carcinoma of the head and neck [corrected]. J Clin Oncol 2009;27(11):1864–71.
29. Machiels JP, Haddad RI, Fayette J, et al. Afatinib versus methotrexate as second-line treatment in patients with recurrent or metastatic squamous-cell carcinoma of the head and neck progressing on or after platinum-based therapy (LUX-Head & Neck 1): an open-label, randomised phase 3 trial. Lancet Oncol 2015;16(5): 583–94.
30. Perisanidis C. Prevalence of EGFR tyrosine kinase domain mutations in head and neck squamous cell carcinoma: cohort study and systematic review. In Vivo 2017;31(1):23–34.
31. Lynch TJ, Bell DW, Sordella R, et al. Activating mutations in the epidermal growth factor receptor underlying responsiveness of non-small-cell lung cancer to gefitinib. N Engl J Med 2004;350(21):2129–39.
32. Zhang J, Saba NF, Chen GZ, et al. Targeting HER (ERBB) signaling in head and neck cancer: an essential update. Mol Aspects Med 2015;45:74–86.
33. Wheeler DL, Huang S, Kruser TJ, et al. Mechanisms of acquired resistance to cetuximab: role of HER (ErbB) family members. Oncogene 2008;27(28):3944–56.
34. Erjala K, Sundvall M, Junttila TT, et al. Signaling via ErbB2 and ErbB3 associates with resistance and epidermal growth factor receptor (EGFR) amplification with sensitivity to EGFR inhibitor gefitinib in head and neck squamous cell carcinoma cells. Clin Cancer Res 2006;12(13):4103–11.
35. Wang D, Qian G, Zhang H, et al. HER3 targeting sensitizes HNSCC to cetuximab by reducing HER3 activity and HER2/HER3 dimerization: evidence from cell line and patient-derived xenograft models. Clin Cancer Res 2017;23(3):677–86.
36. Madoz-Gurpide J, Zazo S, Chamizo C, et al. Activation of MET pathway predicts poor outcome to cetuximab in patients with recurrent or metastatic head and neck cancer. J Transl Med 2015;13:282.
37. Birchmeier C, Birchmeier W, Gherardi E, et al. Met, metastasis, motility and more. Nat Rev Mol Cell Biol 2003;4(12):915–25.
38. Stabile LP, He G, Lui VW, et al. c-Src activation mediates erlotinib resistance in head and neck cancer by stimulating c-Met. Clin Cancer Res 2013;19(2):380–92.
39. Xu H, Stabile LP, Gubish CT, et al. Dual blockade of EGFR and c-Met abrogates redundant signaling and proliferation in head and neck carcinoma cells. Clin Cancer Res 2011;17(13):4425–38.

40. Seiwert TY, Jagadeeswaran R, Faoro L, et al. The MET receptor tyrosine kinase is a potential novel therapeutic target for head and neck squamous cell carcinoma. Cancer Res 2009;69(7):3021–31.
41. Bertotti A, Sassi F. Molecular pathways: sensitivity and resistance to anti-EGFR antibodies. Clin Cancer Res 2015;21(15):3377–83.
42. Huang S, Benavente S, Armstrong EA, et al. p53 modulates acquired resistance to EGFR inhibitors and radiation. Cancer Res 2011;71(22):7071–9.
43. Holz C, Niehr F, Boyko M, et al. Epithelial-mesenchymal-transition induced by EGFR activation interferes with cell migration and response to irradiation and cetuximab in head and neck cancer cells. Radiother Oncol 2011;101(1):158–64.

Anti-PD-1 Immune Checkpoint Blockade for Head and Neck Cancer
Biomarkers of Response and Resistance

Christopher A. Maroun, MD[a,b], Rajarsi Mandal, MD[a,b,*]

KEYWORDS

• Immunotherapy • Checkpoint blockade • Anti-PD-1 • Biomarkers • Response

KEY POINTS

- The evaluation of biomarkers for response and resistance to immune checkpoint blockade is currently an active and rapidly evolving area of research.
- There are multiple molecular and physiologic mechanisms through which head and neck cancers may develop therapeutic resistance to immunotherapy.
- Proposed biomarkers undergoing investigation include tumor mutational burden (TMB), PD-L1 expression, and DNA mismatch repair deficiency.
- A highly precise predictive biomarker for immunotherapy response has yet to be identified.

BACKGROUND

Immunotherapy in recent years has solidified its position as the fourth pillar of cancer treatment alongside surgery, chemotherapy, and radiation. Although in its infancy, when compared with these other conventional therapeutic strategies, immunotherapy has provided a chance for prolonged survival, and in some cases even cure, for patients who previously would have been given a terminal diagnosis. In head and neck cancer in particular, the advent of antiprogrammed cell death protein 1 (anti-PD-1) immune checkpoint blockade has shown modest response rates in patients with recurrent or metastatic mucosal squamous cell carcinoma.[1,2] Additionally, immune checkpoint inhibitors are being explored in the neoadjuvant setting for primary head and neck tumors in multiple trials, either as single agents or in combination with other

[a] Department of Otolaryngology–Head and Neck Surgery, Johns Hopkins University, Baltimore, MD 21287, USA; [b] Bloomberg-Kimmel Institute for Cancer Immunotherapy at Johns Hopkins, Baltimore, MD 21287, USA
* Corresponding author. Department of Otolaryngology–Head and Neck Surgery, Bloomberg-Kimmel Institute for Cancer Immunotherapy at Johns Hopkins, Baltimore, MD 21287.
E-mail address: rmandal6@jhmi.edu

Otolaryngol Clin N Am 54 (2021) 751–759
https://doi.org/10.1016/j.otc.2021.04.006

treatment modalities.[3] Although the data thus far certainly suggest that there is at least a subset of head and neck cancer patients that will greatly benefit from treatment with immune agents, most patients appear to be resistant to immunotherapy. Therefore, one of the greatest challenges within the realm of immunotherapy in its current state is the ability to predict which patients are most likely to benefit from treatment with these agents. Several biomarkers have been proposed within the literature and have been explored within the context of clinical trials, including tumor mutational burden, expression of immune checkpoint ligands, and DNA mismatch repair deficiency, with no single biomarker that has been identified thus far with the ability to accurately and consistently predict response in most cases.[4–6] In this article, the various mechanisms of resistance to immunotherapy and biomarkers of response that have so far been explored in the literature are outlined.

IMMUNE-MEDIATED TUMOR CLEARANCE

At its most basic level, immune-mediated tumor clearance initially requires recognition of the tumor by the immune system. This may occur at the level of the innate immune system, such as through natural killer (NK) cells, which recognize and eradicate cells that do not express autologous HLA molecules on their cell membrane. It may also occur at the level of the adaptive immune system, whereby tumor antigens must be processed and presented to immune cells via HLA molecules on the surface of antigen-presenting cells. This presentation of antigen is usually followed by the engagement of costimulatory molecules that then augment and amplify the immune cascade, leading to activation of T cells and other immune cells. In similar fashion, activation of these immune pathways often results in the development of immune memory, mediated by memory T and B cells that may play a role in the prevention of tumor recurrence and distant metastasis. Therefore, in an ideal situation, immune-mediated tumor clearance may then take place on 2 fronts: locally within the primary tumor bed, and systemically in the form of immune surveillance.

In a situation where there is a chronically present antigen and persistent activation of the immune system, such as in the presence of a tumor or chronic viral infection, immune regulatory pathways are triggered that are meant to prevent overstimulation, as a type of evolutionary safeguard against deleterious autoimmunity.[7] These pathways eventually lead to immune inhibition and homeostasis, through the altered expression of various receptors and ligands on both immune and nonimmune cells. One example of such is the PD-1 receptor, which is upregulated primarily on T cells, and its ligand PD-L1, which is expressed by both tumor cells and other immune cells. When a T cell expresses high levels of PD-1 on its surface above a certain threshold, it assumes an exhausted phenotype, and is no longer an effective mediator of the immune response. By blocking the PD-1/PD-L1 interaction through the use of antibodies, T cells may become invigorated, reactivating the immune response (or slowing the progression toward terminal T cell exhaustion) and potentially leading to a more robust immune surveillance long-term.

MECHANISMS OF RESISTANCE

Theoretically, resistance to immunotherapy may occur at any step along the pathway of immune activation, from the generation of tumor antigen until the initiation of tumor cell death. Although immune checkpoint blockade at its core serves to release the brakes from the immune system, the system still requires an immunologic fuel in order to instigate and maintain an appropriate antitumor response. Some factors that increase a tumor's ability to resist the immune system and therefore immunotherapy are present at baseline; this may be thought of as intrinsic resistance. Other factors of resistance may develop secondary to inflammatory signals that are generated as part of an immune response to the tumor; this may be thought of as adaptive resistance. Understanding the various mechanisms of resistance is important when considering the various biomarker candidates and their limitations, as while a tumor may exhibit certain intrinsic factors that are favorable for response at baseline, that same tumor has the potential for adapting other mechanisms of resistance either during or after therapy.

Antigens that are expressed by tumor cells via genetic tumor mutations are referred to as neoantigens. It has been shown that tumors with higher neoantigen loads have increased CD8+ T cell and cytolytic activity.[8] Increased CD8+ T cell activity has been associated with increased survival in head and neck squamous cell carcinoma.[9] Although neoantigens differ in their binding capabilities and their potency in terms of their individual ability to generate an immune response, in general, it has been demonstrated, that tumors with a higher neoantigen load will respond better to immunotherapy.[10] Additionally, 2 tumors with similar neoantigen loads, but that differ in the quality of their neoantigens, would be expected to display a difference in response. It has been shown that head and neck tumors may differ greatly in their genetic and mutational profiles at baseline.[11] Therefore, the underlying genetic makeup of a particular tumor will likely make it more or less resistant to immunotherapy secondary to the resultant expression of neoantigens. As a testament to this, neoantigen-directed therapies, including neoantigen vaccines and other modalities thought to be synergistic with immune checkpoint blockade, constitute another exciting area of immunotherapy research.[12]

Head and neck tumors have been shown to regularly form neoantigens, similar to other smoking-related cancers in the lung, esophagus, and bladder.[12] However, tumors of the head and neck have also been shown to have other genetic alterations that promote tumor progression and escape from the immune system. Specifically, loss of the ability to actually present antigen is a critically important and regular feature of a significant proportion of head and neck tumors.[13] The antigen presentation machinery consists of multiple different parts of the cell, and genetic alterations affecting any of those parts may result in an inhibition of antigen presentation, which is crucial for immune recognition and subsequent activation. Specifically within head and neck tumors, mutations in interferon signaling pathways, major histocompatibility complex (MHC) class I expression, and transporter associated with antigen processing complex (TAP) 1 and 2 have been reported and are associated with immune evasion.[14–16]

Other than specific genetic alterations, tumor genetic heterogeneity in particular is an interesting concept, as it describes the presence of multiple different subclones of tumor cells within a particular tumor, each harboring different mutations resulting in antigens of varying immunogenicity.[17] Subclones may be preferentially targeted by the immune system, leaving other subclones undetected; this is thought to contribute to instances where a tumor response to treatment is initially observed, but then results in relapse later in time. Tumor heterogeneity in head and neck squamous cell carcinoma has been shown to be associated with decreased survival.[18]

Besides their genetic makeup, different tumors may differ greatly in their immune constitution. Although the two are likely not mutually exclusive, there are multiple other factors that may determine the size and makeup of the immune response. Studies have shown that the composition of the immune infiltrate within the tumor microenvironment prior to treatment with immunotherapy is significantly different between responders and nonresponders. This suggests that there are certain immune elements that may either facilitate or suppress continued immune-mediated tumor clearance in response to checkpoint blockade. In fact, it has been shown in numerous studies that some immune cells and inflammatory pathways are effectively protumorigenic. An example is the presence of M2 macrophages and myeloid-derived suppressor cells (MDSC) commonly found in head and neck squamous tumors, which have been shown to be important sources of immunosuppressive cytokines such as transforming growth factor beta (TGF-b) and interleukin-10 (IL-10).[13] It has been shown that circulating levels of MDSC in melanoma patients treated with ipilimumab are associated with clinical response, suggesting that the pretreatment presence of these immune cells can be used to denote resistance and therefore, in certain contexts, predict response.[19] Although the bulk of immunotherapy research and development thus far has focused on predominantly T-cell targeted therapies, such as anti-PD-1 treatment, the contribution of the myeloid compartment to resistance to therapy, especially in the head and neck, is becoming increasingly important.

BIOMARKERS OF RESPONSE

Immunotherapy has engendered a paradigm shift throughout the field of oncology in the overall treatment strategy for patients with advanced disease. Coupled with the innovative technological advances in the past decade, clinical and scientific efforts have focused on how to better predict response to immune-based therapies. Many of the biomarkers that have been thus far studied are intricately related to the mechanisms of resistance that have been outlined previously. Further, as a higher level of granularity is achieved by defining how different immune pathways may become dominant within each individual tumor, the unearthing of new biomarkers may hold more utility than simply identifying responders from nonresponders. Rather, the use of biomarkers to guide therapeutic selection, especially given the vast array of immune agents that are currently being developed, will be inherently vital as a new era of personalized oncology begins.

Programmed Cell Death Protein 1 Expression

Perhaps the most well-known and earliest biomarker of response to immunotherapy, specifically with PD-1 blockade, is the tissue expression of its primary ligand, PD-L1. PD-L1 expression within the tumor microenvironment may be present as a result of multiple mechanisms, as well as in numerous histologic configurations. It has been shown that certain oncogenic molecular pathways that contribute to malignant cell proliferation and tumor progression may also contribute to local immunosuppression through the upregulation of PD-L1.[7] For example, some lymphomas and types of lung cancer exhibit constitutive activation of anaplastic lymphoma kinase (ALK), which leads to baseline expression of PD-L1 as a result of signal transducer and activator of transcription 3 (STAT3) signaling.[20] This constitutive expression of PD-L1 by tumor cells themselves can be easily visualized through immunohistochemistry (IHC) staining, and is an example of intrinsic immune resistance.[7] In contrast, PD-L1 expression may be induced on the surface of cancer cells as a result of inflammatory mediators that are released during an antitumor immune response. Specifically, interferon-gamma (IFN-g), which is a key inflammatory cytokine and marker of immune activation, is known to be a strong inducer of PD-L1 expression.[21] IFN-g is produced by several immune cell types, including natural killers, CD4+ and CD8+ T cells, and natural killer T cells.[22] Although generally considered as having proimmune functionality, IFN-g may also contribute to adaptive immune resistance within the tumor bed secondary to its ability to cause induced PD-L1 expression on tumor cells in an effort to maintain immune homeostasis. Other inflammatory cytokines that have been shown to contribute to induced PD-L1 expression include IL-1a, IL-10, IL-27, and IL-32g.[23]

Clinically, PD-L1 was first described as a biomarker of response to immunotherapy in the earliest trials of anti-PD-1 therapy in advanced melanoma, nonsmall cell lung cancer, castration-resistant prostate cancer, renal cell carcinoma, and colorectal cancer.[6] In a previous study by Topalian and colleagues, 296 patients were treated with anti-PD-1 antibody and stratified into responders and nonresponders according to modified RECIST criteria. Tumors from 42 patients were then analyzed for PD-L1 positivity with a 5% expression threshold using immunohistochemistry. The investigators found that none of the 17 patients with PD-L1 negative tumors had an objective response, compared with 9 of 25 patients with PD-L1 positive tumors who did have an objective response. This initial work highlights the importance of assessing PD-L1 as a valuable, albeit imperfect, biomarker for patient selection for treatment with immunotherapy.

In head and neck cancers, 2 important clinical trials that have assessed clinical efficacy of the anti-PD-1 agents nivolumab and pembrolizumab are Checkmate-141 and KEYNOTE-012, respectively.[24,25] In both of these trials, PD-L1 positivity was defined as greater than 1% expression and was associated with significant improvements in overall survival when compared with patients who were PD-L1 negative. The prevalence of PD-L1 expression in head and neck cancers based on IHC staining varies depending on the detection antibody and cutoff used, with rates in the literature being reported between 31% and 66%.[26] Additionally, head and neck cancers in particular posit an additional variable that has been shown to affect PD-L1 expression: HPV status. HPV-positive tumors have been shown to exhibit a much higher rate of PD-L1 positivity compared with their HPV-negative counterparts, up to 70% compared with only 29% in 1 study.[27] Despite the obvious correlation between PD-L1 expression and immunotherapy response, the fact remains that most patients with PD-L1 positive tumors do not respond, demonstrating its potential shortcomings as a biomarker.

Tumor Mutational Burden

As previously discussed, the genetic landscape of any particular tumor influences the composition and strength of its associated immune response. Other than contributing to intrinsic resistance through the promotion of immunosuppressive pathways and signals, mutations leading to the expression of immunogenic neoantigens are thought to be a major driving force in the propagation of immune-mediated tumor clearance through antigen-specific cytolytic activity. The clinical utility of tumor mutational burden (TMB) as a biomarker of response to immunotherapy was first demonstrated in patients with melanoma who were treated with ipilimumab or tremelimumab, antibody antagonists of cytotoxic T-lymphocyte associated antigen 4 (CTLA-4), another inhibitory immune checkpoint receptor.[28] In this study of 64 patients, high mutational load was associated with clinical benefit, including prolonged survival. Importantly however, the authors noted the presence of patients with high mutational load who did not respond to therapy, indicating, similar to PD-L1, that high TMB alone is insufficient in ensuring durable clinical benefit.

Since the association between TMB and response to immunotherapy was first discovered, the understanding of the relationship between the two has been refined. High TMB is associated with immunotherapy response secondary to the resultant generation of immunogenic neoantigens. However, the discordance arises in situations where the total number of mutations does not reflect the absolute number of immunogenic mutations. Specifically, it has been shown that insertion/deletion mutations, which are far more likely to result in frameshifts leading to neoantigen formation, are an important driver of response to immunotherapy.[29] These frameshifting mutations can generate large numbers of immunogenic peptides that can elicit immune-mediated tumor clearance. Although nonsense mediated decay can help to limit the expression of these aberrant proteins, many do indeed generate immune responses. More recently, whole-exome sequencing data used to quantify TMB has been merged with transcriptomic data to identify mutations specifically within expressed genes, which have been found to be a better predictor of response than TMB alone.[30] In head and neck tumors, tumor mutational burden has been found to be a positive predictive biomarker for response to checkpoint inhibitors in several studies.[31–33]

DNA Mismatch Repair Deficiency

Related to mutational burden, and certainly an important predictor of response to immunotherapy, is DNA mismatch repair deficiency (MMR-d). MMR-d is a well-studied cause of genetic instability, classically associated with the development of colorectal cancer.[34] MMR-d leads to expansions of tandem repetitive segments of DNA termed microsatellites that lead to instability in that region of DNA. MMR-d also promotes the subsequent development of a large number of frameshifting mutations in tumor DNA. Consequently, MMR-d tumors have been shown to be highly responsive to immunotherapy, leading to the historic approval by the US Food and Drug Administration (FDA) for use of anti-PD-1 therapy for all metastatic or unresectable solid tumors with microsatellite instability, the first time a therapy has been approved regardless of the tissue type.[35] It has been recently demonstrated that a significant contributor in response to immunotherapy in MMR-d tumors is largely driven by insertion/deletion (indel) mutational load, which MMR-d tumors are much more likely to develop.[36] The utility of MMR-d as a biomarker of response in the head and neck, however, appears to be limited, as the proportion of head and neck tumors with MMR-d is not particularly high.[37] In addition, head and neck squamous cell carcinoma ranks somewhat average in terms of its indel mutation load, which reflects a lesser involvement of this mutational process in the disease process.[29]

HPV Status

Being virally driven, HPV-positive head and neck tumors provide an incredibly interesting platform for immunotherapy research given the extra element that viral antigens potentially bring to the stage. HPV-positive tumors are already established as a distinct entity from their HPV-negative counterparts clinically, genetically, and molecularly, so it is no surprise that their interaction with the immune system is similarly unique.[11] HPV-positive head and neck squamous cell carcinoma (HNSCC) has been shown to be among the most highly immune infiltrated cancers, and shows increased intratumoral cytolytic immune activity compared with HPV-negative HNSCC.[9] It has been hypothesized that HPV-positive tumors, therefore, are poised to be far more responsive to immune checkpoint blockade compared with HPV-negative tumors; however, the data thus far have been conflicting.[38]

Although initial results from KEYNOTE-012 demonstrated an increased objective response rate (ORR) to pembrolizumab in HPV-positive tumors, results from KEYNOTE-040 failed to corroborate this.[25,39] Similarly, CHECKMATE-141 did not generate any significant difference in ORR between HPV-positive and HPV-negative patients treated with nivolumab.[2] It is possible that other confounding factors affecting immunotherapy response may contribute to the variability in results seen from these and other trials. Interestingly, other biomarkers of response appear to have differential utility in HPV-positive and HPV-negative tumors. For example, TMB in particular appears to be less predictive in HPV-positive tumors compared with HPV-negative tumors.[33] In fact, in 1 study, despite showing similar response rates between HPV-negative and HPV-positive HNSCC treated with anti-PD-1/PD-L1 agents,

HPV-positive tumors were shown to have a significantly lower TMB.[31] This is striking, and illustrates the potential influence of viral antigens on immunotherapy response independent of mutation-associated neoantigens. Collectively, however, based on the currently available data, it remains unlikely that HPV status alone can be used as a biomarker of response, and it will likely need to be combined with other factors to increase its utility.

SUMMARY

Although immunotherapy has expanded the armamentarium of therapeutic options for patients with advanced disease, significant strides have yet to be achieved to improve overall response rates. Despite understanding of the various mechanisms of resistance, cancer is an ever-changing entity, with the ability to disguise itself, adapt, and mutate, in order to evade therapy. Although the most well-studied biomarkers of response have been outlined here, there remain dozens of other potential biomarkers that have been proposed and are under investigation, some as relatively simple as smoking-related gene signatures, and others more complex, utilizing multi-omic computational analyses to discover gene signature panels and other tumor features associated with response. The ideal sought after biomarker would be simple to query, provide results quickly (in order to be most clinically useful), and be cost-effective. However, the most useful biomarker for predicting response in the future is more likely to constitute a combination of markers in order to make the most of the understanding of the complex interaction between cancer and the immune system.

CLINICS CARE POINTS

- Currently available biomarkers that have been studied and may have clinical utility in the head and neck include TMB and PD-L1 expression and DNA mismatch repair deficiency.
- HPV-positive tumors may be more responsive to immune checkpoint blockade; however; further data are needed to fully ascertain any potential correlation.

DISCLOSURE

The authors have nothing to disclose.

REFERENCES

1. Mehra R, Seiwert TY, Gupta S, et al. Efficacy and safety of pembrolizumab in recurrent/metastatic head and neck squamous cell carcinoma: pooled analyses after long-term follow-up in KEYNOTE-012. Br J Cancer 2018;119(2):153–9.
2. Ferris RL, Blumenschein G Jr, Fayette J, et al. Nivolumab vs investigator's choice in recurrent or metastatic squamous cell carcinoma of the head and neck: 2-year long-term survival update of CheckMate 141 with analyses by tumor PD-L1 expression. Oral Oncol 2018;81:45–51.
3. Stafford M, Kaczmar J. The neoadjuvant paradigm reinvigorated: a review of pre-surgical immunotherapy in HNSCC. Cancers Head Neck 2020;5:4.
4. Rizvi NA, Hellman MD, Snyder A, et al. Cancer immunology. Mutational landscape determines sensitivity to PD-1 blockade in non-small cell lung cancer. Science 2015;348:124–8.

5. Le DT, Durham JN, Smith KN, et al. Mismatch repair deficiency predicts response of solid tumors to PD-1 blockade. Science 2017;357:409–13.
6. Topalian SL, Hodi FS, Brahmer JR, et al. Safety, activity, and immune correlates of anti-PD-1 antibody in cancer. N Engl J Med 2012;366:2443–54.
7. Pardoll DM. The blockade of immune checkpoints in cancer immunotherapy. Nat Rev Cancer 2012;12(4):252–64.
8. Thorsson V, Gibbs DL, Brown SD, et al. The immune landscape of cancer. Immunity 2018;48:812–30.
9. Mandal R, Senbabaoglu Y, Desrichard A, et al. The head and neck cancer immune landscape and its immunotherapeutic implications. JCI Insight 2016; 1(17):e89829.
10. Rizvi NA, Hellmann MD, Snyder A, et al. Mutational landscape determines sensitivity to PD-1 blockade in non-small cell lung cancer. Science 2015;348(6230): 124–8.
11. The Cancer Genome Atlas Network. Comprehensive genomic characterization of head and neck squamous cell carcinoma. Nature 2015;517:576–82.
12. Schumacher TN, Schreiber RD. Neoantigens in cancer immunotherapy. Science 2015;348(6230):69–74.
13. Lee MY, Allen CT. Mechanisms of resistance to T cell-based immunotherapy in head and neck cancer. Head Neck 2020;42:2722–33.
14. López-Albaitero A, Nayak JV, Ogino T, et al. Role of antigen processing machinery in the in vitro resistance of squamous cell carcinoma of the head and neck cells to recognition by CTL. J Immunol 2006;176(6):3402–9.
15. Meissner M, Reichert TE, Kunkel M, et al. Defects in the human leukocyte antigen class I antigen processing machinery in head and neck squamous cell carcinoma: association with clinical outcome. Clin Cancer Res 2005;11(7):2552–60.
16. Sharma P, Hu-Lieskovan S, Wargo JA, et al. Primary, adaptive and acquired resistance to cancer immunotherapy. Cell 2017;168(4):707–23.
17. Gerlinger M, Rowan AJ, Horswell S, et al. Intratumor heterogeneity and branched evolution revealed by multiregion sequencing. N Engl J Med 2012;366(10): 883–92.
18. Mroz EA, Tward AM, Hammon RJ, et al. Intratumor genetic heterogeneity and mortality in head and neck cancer: analysis of data from the cancer genome atlas. PLoS Med 2015;12(2):e1001786.
19. Weber R, Fleming V, Hu X, et al. Myeloid-derived suppressor cells hinder the anticancer activity of immune checkpoint inhibitors. Front Immunol 2018;9:1310.
20. Marzec M, Zhang Q, Goradia A, et al. Oncogenic kinase NPM/ALK induces through STAT3 expression of immunosuppressive protein CD274 (PD-L1, B7-H1). Proc Natl Acad Sci U S A 2008;105:20852–7.
21. Scognamiglio T, Chen YT. Beyond the percentages of PD-L1-positive tumor cells: induced versus constitutive PD-L1 expression in primary and metastatic head and neck squamous cell carcinoma. Head Neck Pathol 2018;12:221–9.
22. Wilke CM, Wei S, Wang L, et al. Dual biological effects of the cytokines interleukin-10 and interferon-g. Cancer Immunol Immunother 2011;60:1529–41.
23. Chen S, Crabill GA, Pritchard TS, et al. Mechanisms regulating PD-L1 expression on tumor and immune cells. J Immunother Cancer 2019;7:305.
24. Ferris RL, Blumenschein G Jr, Fayette J, et al. Nivolumab for recurrent squamous-cell carcinoma of the head and neck. N Engl J Med 2016;375:1856–67.
25. Chow LQ, Haddad R, Gupta S, et al. Antitumor activity of pembrolizumab in biomarker-unselected patients with recurrent and/or metastatic head and neck

squamous cell carcinoma: results from the phase Ib KEYNOTE-012 expansion cohort. J Clin Oncol 2016;34:3838–45.
26. Patel SP, Kurzrock R. PD-L1 expression as a predictive biomarker in cancer immunotherapy. Mol Cancer Ther 2015;14(4):847–56.
27. Lyford-Pike S, Peng S, Young GD, et al. Evidence for a role of the PD-1:PD-L1 pathway in immune resistance of HPV-associated head and neck squamous cell carcinoma. Cancer Res 2013;73(6):1733–41.
28. Snyder A, Makarov V, Merghoub T, et al. Genetic basis for clinical response to CTLA-4 blockade in melanoma. N Engl J Med 2014;371(23):2189–99.
29. Turajlic S, Litchfield K, Xu H, et al. Insertion-and-deletion-derived tumour-specific neoantigens and the immunogenic phenotype: a pan-cancer analysis. Lancet 2017;8(18):P1009–21.
30. Anagnostou V, Bruhm DC, Niknafs N, et al. Integrative tumor and immune cell multi-omic analyses predict response to immune checkpoint blockade in melanoma. Cell Rep Med 2020;1(8):100139.
31. Hanna GJ, Lizotte P, Cavanaugh M, et al. Frameshift events predict antiPD-1/L1 response in head and neck cancer. JCI Insight 2018;3(4):e98811.
32. Haddad RI, Seiwert TY, Chow LQM, et al. Genomic determinants of response to pembrolizumab in head and neck squamous cell carcinoma (HNSCC). J Clin Oncol 2017;35(Suppl 15):6009.
33. Seiwert TY, et al. Biomarkers predictive of response to pembrolizumab in head and neck cancer (HNSCC). Abstract 339. AACR Annual Meeting 2018. Chicago, April 14-18, 2018.
34. Poulogiannis G, Frayling IM, Arends MJ. DNA mismatch repair deficiency in sporadic colorectal cancer and Lynch syndrome. Histopathology 2010;56(2):167–79.
35. U.S. Food and Drug Administration. FDA approves first cancer treatment for any solid tumor with a specific genetic feature. Silver Spring: FDA News Release; 2017.
36. Mandal R, Samstein RM, Lee KW, et al. Genetic diversity of tumors with mismatch repair deficiency influences anti-PD-1 immunotherapy response. Science 2019; 364:485–91.
37. Cilona M, Locatello LG, Novelli L, et al. The mismatch repair system (MMR) in head and neck carcinogenesis and its role in modulating the response to immunotherapy: a critical review. Cancers (Basel) 2020;12(10):3006.
38. Oliva M, Spreafico A, Taberna M, et al. Immune biomarkers of response to immune-checkpoint inhibitors in head and neck squamous cell carcinoma. Ann Oncol 2019;30:57–67.
39. Soulieres D, Cohen E, Le Tourneau C, et al. Updated survival results of the KEYNOTE-040 study of pembrolizumab vs standard-of-care chemotherapy for recurrent or metastatic head and neck squamous cell carcinoma. Abstract Cancer Res 2018;CT115.

Advances in Adoptive Cell Therapy for Head and Neck Cancer

Scott M. Norberg, DO[a,*], Christian S. Hinrichs, MD[b]

KEYWORDS

- Adoptive cell therapy • Chimeric antigen receptor • T-cell receptor
- Tumor-infiltrating lymphocyte • Oropharyngeal squamous cell carcinoma
- Human papillomavirus • Head and neck cancer

KEY POINTS

- Tumor-infiltrating lymphocyte and gene-engineered T-cell receptor T-cell therapy targeting human papilloma virus (HPV) viral antigens have each demonstrated the ability to induce tumor regression in patients with HPV-associated epithelial cancer including head and neck cancer.
- Tumor-intrinsic defects in genes important for antigen presentation and interferon response seem to portend resistance to adoptively transferred T cells and may be overcome by earlier treatment with adoptive cell therapy (ACT).
- One approach to enhance the function of adoptively transferred T cells with membrane-tethered cytokines is being explored.
- Further clinical advances using ACT in head and neck cancer may come through targeting of non-HPV antigens including Epstein-Barr virus viral proteins and cancer germline antigens.

INTRODUCTION

Adoptive cell therapy (ACT) is a promising new treatment modality that has demonstrated clinical activity in hematologic cancers and a subset of solid tumors. The most clinically successful type of ACT thus far has been chimeric antigen receptor (CAR) T-cell therapy. CAR T-cell therapies targeting the lineage-restricted antigen CD19 have been approved by the US Food and Drug Administration (FDA) for the treatment of B cell malignancies.[1–3] CAR T cells express synthetic receptors that engage target antigens on the surface of tumor cells. Clinical application of CAR

[a] Genitourinary Malignancy Branch, National Cancer Institute, 10 Center Drive, Room 3-3132, Bethesda, MD 20892, USA; [b] Genitourinary Malignancy Branch, National Cancer Institute, 10 Center Drive, Room 4B04, Bethesda, MD 20892, USA
* Corresponding author.
E-mail address: scott.norberg@nih.gov

Otolaryngol Clin N Am 54 (2021) 761–768
https://doi.org/10.1016/j.otc.2021.05.001
oto.theclinics.com

T-cell therapy has thus far been limited to hematologic malignancies because of the lack of cell surface antigens that can be safely targeted in solid tumors.[4,5] Early studies targeting cell surface antigens in solid tumors with CAR T cells resulted in significant toxicity through targeting of vital healthy tissue. A previous study testing CAR T-cell therapy targeting carbonic anhydrase IX in patients with metastatic renal cell carcinoma led to significant on-target, off-tumor toxicity.[6,7] Careful selection of target antigen is necessary to apply this therapy to common epithelial cancers like head and neck cancer.[5]

Tumor-infiltrating lymphocyte (TIL) and gene-engineered T-cell receptor (TCR) T-cell therapies have demonstrated clinical activity in a subset of solid cancers. TIL and TCR T-cell therapy have the advantage of targeting antigens that are from proteins residing inside of the cell or on the cell surface. Therefore, a broad range of tumor-specific antigens can be targeted with highly potent T cells with minimal to no targeting of vital healthy tissue. In TIL therapy, autologous tumor-specific T cells are harvested from resected metastatic tumor deposits. The natural T cells are expanded ex vivo to large quantities and administered back to the patient by intravenous infusion. These T cells have been shown to target mutated neoantigens, cancer germline antigens, and viral antigens expressed by cancer cells.[8,9] TIL therapy has its foundation in the successful treatment of metastatic melanoma.[10] Gene-engineered TCR T-cell therapy involves isolation of peripheral blood lymphocytes by apheresis. These T cells are then genetically engineered to express a high-affinity TCR that recognizes a peptide from a tumor antigen in the context of a specific HLA molecule. Early studies with TCR T-cell therapy targeting the cancer germline antigen New York esophageal squamous cell carcinoma-1 (NY-ESO-1) demonstrated clinical activity in patients with synovial cell sarcoma and melanoma.[11] Recent clinical studies testing TIL and TCR-T cell therapy in treatment-refractory human papilloma virus (HPV)-positive epithelial cancers including head and neck cancer demonstrated clinical activity in the last-line setting.[12–14]

ADVANCES IN ADOPTIVE T-CELL THERAPY IN HEAD AND NECK CANCER

HPV-associated oropharyngeal cancer is a common type of head and neck cancer that harbors viral antigens that can be targeted by ACT.[15,16] These viral antigens are ideal target antigens for T-cell therapy, because they are not present in vital healthy tissue, important for the transformation and survival of cancer cells, and constitutively expressed by cancer cells.[17,18] T cells targeting the viral antigens E6 and E7 have been identified in tumor-infiltrating lymphocytes from cervical cancer specimens, and better clinical outcomes have been associated with T cell reactivity against these antigens, indicating that ACT with HPV-specific T cells may be an effective treatment for HPV-associated cancers.[19,20]

The first attempt to target these antigens with adoptively transferred T cells was with TIL therapy. In a phase II clinical trial, patients with HPV-associated epithelial cancers were treated with autologous TIL generated preferentially from T cell subcultures reactive toward the E6 and E7 viral antigens.[13] Patients received a conditioning chemotherapy regimen of cyclophosphamide 60 mg/kg for 2 days and fludarabine 25 mg/m^2 for 5 days followed by a single infusion of TIL and high-dose aldesleukin. Objective tumor responses were seen in 5 of 18 (28%) patients with cervical cancer and 2 of 11 (18%) patients with other HPV-positive cancers including head and neck. Two of the responses in patients with cervical cancer were complete and have been ongoing now for more than 6 years. One of 5 patients with HPV-associated head and neck cancer had an objective response. The patient was a 60-year-old man with squamous cell carcinoma of the tonsil. He was previously treated with 6 systemic anticancer agents and had multiple thoracic metastases that were progressing prior to therapy. Following treatment, he had complete regression of his thoracic disease. He subsequently developed new brain metastases that were resected. He has been without evidence of disease now for more than 5 years. Exploratory analysis from this trial demonstrated that administered TILs displaying a greater frequency of HPV-reactive T cells (as measured by the frequency of T cells responding to E6 and E7 peptide stimulation) and higher concentrations of HPV-specific interferon (IFN)-γ release correlated with response. Furthermore, the frequency of HPV-reactive T cells in peripheral blood 1 month after treatment correlated positively with clinical response.[13] Viral and nonviral antigens were targeted by the TIL administered to the 2 patients who had complete tumor regression.[12] Based on these results, a multicenter, multicohort, nonrandomized, industry-sponsored trial is being conducted to test TIL therapy (LN-145) in patients with recurrent and metastatic squamous cell carcinoma of the head and neck (NCT03083873).

Gene-engineered TCR T-cell therapy is a next-generation approach to ACT that does not require surgery and creates a cell therapy product with well-defined specificity toward a target antigen. A TCR targeting the HPV16 $E6_{29\text{-}38}$-peptide presented in the context of HLA-A*02:01 was discovered from the tumor-infiltrating lymphocyte in a patient with metastatic HPV16-associated anal cancer.[21] A first-in-human, single-center, phase I/II study was then conducted using this TCR in patients with metastatic HPV16-associated epithelial cancer.[14] In this study, patients received a conditioning chemotherapy regimen followed by a single infusion of autologous peripheral blood T cells genetically engineered to express the HLA-A*02:01-restricted, HPV16 $E6_{29\text{-}38}$-specific TCR (E6 TCR-T cells) and high-dose aldesleukin administered to patient tolerance. The starting dose of cells was 1 x 10^9, and the highest cell dose was 1-2 x 10^{11}. Twelve patients were treated (1 patient with head and neck cancer). No autoimmune toxicities or DLTs were observed. There were no acute toxicities associated with cell infusion, and no cytokine storm occurred at any dose level. Two of 12 patients (2 of 9 patients at the highest cell dose) attained objective tumor responses. One patient with metastatic anal squamous cell carcinoma who was previously treated with 5 systemic anticancer agents including TIL therapy experienced a partial response, with complete regression of 1 lung tumor and partial regression of 2 lung tumors. The remaining 2 lung tumors were resected at the time of progression. She has been without evidence of disease now for more than 4 years. All patients demonstrated high levels of peripheral blood engraftment with E6 TCR-T cells following treatment (median 30%, range 4% to 53%). The number of infused E6-reactive T cells did not correlate with response.[14] This study demonstrated the ability of TCR T-cell therapy to mediate regression of metastatic HPV-associated cancers.

The clinical testing of E6 TCR-T cells was followed by the discovery of a HPV16 E7-specific, HLA-A*02:01-restricted TCR from an infiltrating lymphocyte in a uterine cervix biopsy from a woman with cervical intraepithelial neoplasia.[22] This TCR (E7 TCR) displayed higher functional avidity than the E6 TCR with the ability to recognize cognate peptide at concentrations as low as 10 pmol.[22] The E7 epitope targeted by this TCR was also found to be highly conserved across different strains of HPV16.[23] A phase I clinical trial was conducted testing the E7 TCR in patients with metastatic HPV16-associated cancers. Twelve patients were treated (4 with head and neck cancer), with 6 patients having objective tumor response. These responses included regression of bulky tumors and complete elimination of some tumors in patients. Four of these responses were in patients with disease refractory to PD-1 inhibitors.

There were 2 responses in patients with head and neck cancer. One response was in a 65-year-old man with metastatic squamous cell carcinoma of the oropharynx with tumors in the lungs, pleura, mediastinum, abdominal wall, retroperitoneum, and bone who was previously treated with 6 systemic anticancer agents including a PD-1 inhibitor and TIL therapy.[24] This study demonstrated the ability of E7 TCR T cells to mediate regression of treatment-refractory, widely metastatic epithelial cancers including PD-1 refractory head and neck cancer. An ongoing phase II clinical trial is currently underway at the National Cancer Institute (NCI) Genitourinary Malignancies Branch to further assess the clinical activity of the E7 TCR (NCT02858310).

FUTURE OF ADOPTIVE T-CELL THERAPY FOR HUMAN PAPILLOMA VIRUS-ASSOCIATED HEAD AND NECK CANCER

The TCR T-cell trials in HPV-associated cancers provide a unique model of studying mechanisms of response and resistance by having constrained variation in both T-cell antigen-targeting and tumor antigen expression. Investigation of T-cell factors in these studies did not provide clear insight into mechanisms of treatment failure. However, the investigation of tumor factors revealed tumor-intrinsic defects in antigen presentation and INF response that demonstrated clear mechanisms of tumor resistance. In the clinical trial testing E6 TCR-T cells, 1 tumor from a patient who did not have a response to therapy was found to have loss of HLA-A*02:01, the antigen presentation molecule required for E6 TCR T-cell recognition of cognate peptide. Another tumor from a patient who did not respond to therapy revealed a truncating mutation in INF-gamma receptor 1, a crucial molecule for tumor sensitivity to T cells. In contrast, a tumor from a patient who did respond to therapy did not have these defects.[14] Similarly, in the clinical trial testing E7 TCR-T cells, 3 resistant tumors demonstrated genetic defects in either HLA-A*02:01 or B2M (necessary components of the E7 TCR target complex), and 1 tumor demonstrated copy loss with decreased expression of genes important for antigen presentation and IFN response including TAP1, TAP2, IFNGR1, and IFNGR2. Three sensitive tumors did not show genetic defects encoding these molecules. These findings suggest that tumors acquire somatic mutations and copy loss defects that confer resistance to T cell-mediated tumor engagement and effector function.[24] Awareness of the development of immune resistance, especially as cancers evolve over time and through multiple therapies, is driving a movement in oncology toward earlier application of immunotherapy including adoptive T-cell therapy.[25,26] A clinical trial at the NCI Genitourinary Malignancies Branch will test E7 TCR-T cell therapy in stage II/III HPV16-positive oropharyngeal cancer in the induction setting (NCT04015336).

Another approach to increase the efficacy of adoptive T-cell therapy is to combine administration of tumor-specific T cells with cytokines such as interleukin-12 (IL-12), which is a potent activator of the innate and adaptive immune system.[27,28] Unfortunately, systemic administration of IL-12 as a single agent can result in significant toxicity.[29] One strategy is to preferentially localize IL-12 to the tumor through genetic engineering of tumor-specific T cells. Toward this end, a clinical trial treating patients with metastatic melanoma using autologous TIL genetically engineered to secrete IL-12 was conducted. Clinical activity was seen even at low doses of adoptively transferred T cells, but severe IL-12-related toxicity limited the development of this approach.[30] A potentially safer approach has been developed where IL-12 is tethered to the membrane of adoptively transferred T cells using a transmembrane anchor domain. In preclinical mouse models of cancer, adoptively transferred T cells expressing membrane-tethered IL-12 demonstrated increased antitumor efficacy, low circulating levels of IL-12 and IFN-γ, and no weight loss indicating a lack of systemic toxicity.[31]

ADOPTIVE T-CELL THERAPY FOR NONHUMAN PAPILLOMA VIRUS-ASSOCIATED HEAD AND NECK CANCER

Epstein-Barr Virus (EBV) has been linked to the development of a subset of head and neck cancers and expresses viral proteins that are ideal targets for adoptive T-cell therapy.[5] Adoptive T-cell therapy with EBV-specific cytotoxic T lymphocytes (CTLs) has been studied for decades as a treatment for EBV after transplantation lymphoproliferative disorder occurring after allogenic hematopoietic stem cell transplantation.[32,33] Clinical trials are testing EBV-specific CTL therapy in patients with EBV-associated nasopharyngeal carcinoma (NCT03769467,NCT02578641). A limitation of EBV-specific CTL therapy is the variable level of T-cell avidity toward the target antigen. In an attempt to consistently target EBV antigens with a significantly large quantity of high-affinity EBV-specific T cells, an active area of investigation is the discovery of high-avidity TCRs targeting EBV viral antigens that could then be tested in patients with EBV-associated diseases such as nasopharyngeal carcinoma.[34]

Cancer germline (CG) antigens are another group of antigens that are rationale targets for ACT. CG antigens are normally expressed by germ cells but can also be expressed by cancer cells. Because germ cells lack expression of MHC class I molecules, they are unable to be recognized by TCRs. Testis-restricted and certain testis-selective CG antigens are rational targets for TCR-T cell therapy.[5] CG antigens have been successfully targeted using TCR T-cell therapy in patients with synovial cell sarcoma and melanoma.[11] Melanoma-associated antigen 4 (MAGE-A4) is a member of a gene family of MAGE proteins. Expression is thought to be restricted to immune-privileged sites and has been found to be expressed in head and neck cancer.[35,36] A clinical trial is testing this TCR in patients with multiple different cancers including head and neck (NCT03132922). Other MAGE protein family members may also be appropriate targets for ACT in head and neck cancer.[37]

Another CG antigen that may be a target for ACT in head and neck cancer is Kita-Kyushu lung cancer antigen 1 (KK-LC-1). KK-LC-1 (encoded by CT83) is a CG antigen that has been reported to have restricted expression in germ cells and in certain epithelial cancers including lung, gastric, breast, and head and neck.[38–40] A TCR targeting KK-LC-1 was identified from the tumor-infiltrating lymphocyte of a patient with metastatic cervical cancer who had a complete response to TIL therapy.[12,40] The single KK-LC-1 TCR clonotype was the dominate clone in the TIL infusion cell product, comprising 67% of the infused T cells. This TCR clonotype was also present at high levels following TIL therapy, suggesting that it might have contributed to cancer regression in this patient.[12] Preclinical studies demonstrated the ability of T cells genetically engineered to express the KK-LC-1 TCR to mediate regression of KK-LC-1 positive epithelial cancers.[40] These findings support the clinical testing of KK-LC-1 TCR-T cells in patients with KK-LC-1 expressing epithelial cancers including head and neck cancer.

SUMMARY

The potential for durable regression of highly refractory tumors makes adoptive T-cell therapy a promising treatment modality for head and neck cancer. Recent success of TIL and gene-engineered TCR-T cell therapy in HPV-associated cancers including head and neck highlight the ability of this therapy to treat advanced epithelial cancers. Strategies to overcome tumor-intrinsic mechanisms of resistance to ACT are being investigated. Further clinical advances using ACT in head and neck cancer may come through targeting of non-HPV antigens including EBV viral proteins and CG antigens.

REFERENCES

1. Neelapu SS, Locke FL, Bartlett NL, et al. Axicabtagene ciloleucel CAR T-cell therapy in refractory large B-cell lymphoma. N Engl J Med 2017;377(26):2531–44.
2. Maude SL, Laetsch TW, Buechner J, et al. . Tisagenlecleucel in children and young adults with B-cell lymphoblastic leukemia. N Engl J Med 2018;378(5): 439–48.
3. Wang M, Munoz J, Goy A, et al. KTE-X19 CAR T-cell therapy in relapsed or refractory mantle-cell lymphoma. N Engl J Med 2020;382(14):1331–42.
4. Leko V, Rosenberg SA. Identifying and targeting human tumor antigens for T cell-based immunotherapy of solid tumors. Cancer Cell 2020;38(4):454–72.
5. Hinrichs CS, Restifo NP. Reassessing target antigens for adoptive T-cell therapy. Nat Biotechnol 2013;31(11):999–1008.
6. Lamers CH, Sleijfer S, Vulto AG, et al. Treatment of metastatic renal cell carcinoma with autologous T-lymphocytes genetically retargeted against carbonic anhydrase IX: first clinical experience. J Clin Oncol 2006;24(13):e20–2.
7. Lamers CH, Sleijfer S, van Steenbergen S,, et al. Treatment of metastatic renal cell carcinoma with CAIX CAR-engineered T cells: clinical evaluation and management of on-target toxicity. Mol Ther 2013;21(4):904–12.
8. Stevanovic S, Draper LM, Langhan MM,, et al. . Complete regression of metastatic cervical cancer after treatment with human papillomavirus-targeted tumor-infiltrating T cells. J Clin Oncol 2015;33(14):1543–50.
9. Zacharakis N, Chinnasamy H, Black M,, et al. Immune recognition of somatic mutations leading to complete durable regression in metastatic breast cancer. Nat Med 2018;24(6):724–30.
10. Goff SL, Dudley ME, Citrin DE,, et al. Randomized, prospective evaluation comparing intensity of lymphodepletion before adoptive transfer of tumor-infiltrating lymphocytes for patients with metastatic melanoma. J Clin Oncol 2016;34(20):2389–97.
11. Robbins PF, Kassim SH, Tran TL,, et al. A pilot trial using lymphocytes genetically engineered with an NY-ESO-1-reactive T-cell receptor: long-term follow-up and correlates with response. Clin Cancer Res 2015;21(5):1019–27.
12. Stevanovic S, Pasetto A, Helman SR,, et al. . Landscape of immunogenic tumor antigens in successful immunotherapy of virally induced epithelial cancer. Science 2017;356(6334):200–5.
13. Stevanovic S, Helman SR, Wunderlich JR,, et al. A phase II study of tumor-infiltrating lymphocyte therapy for human papillomavirus-associated epithelial cancers. Clin Cancer Res 2019;25(5):1486–93.
14. Doran SL, Stevanovic S, Adhikary S, et al. . T-cell receptor gene therapy for human papillomavirus-associated epithelial cancers: a first-in-human, phase I/II study. J Clin Oncol 2019;37(30):2759–68.
15. Viens LJ, Henley SJ, Watson M, et al. Human papillomavirus-associated cancers - United States, 2008-2012. MMWR Morb Mortal Wkly Rep 2016;65(26):661–6.
16. Berman TA, Schiller JT. Human papillomavirus in cervical cancer and oropharyngeal cancer: One cause, two diseases. Cancer 2017;123(12):2219–29.
17. Magaldi TG, Almstead LL, Bellone S, et al. Primary human cervical carcinoma cells require human papillomavirus E6 and E7 expression for ongoing proliferation. Virology 2012;422(1):114–24.

18. Moody CA, Laimins LA. Human papillomavirus oncoproteins: pathways to transformation. Nat Rev Cancer 2010;10(8):550–60.
19. Heusinkveld M, Welters MJ, van Poelgeest MI, et al. The detection of circulating human papillomavirus-specific T cells is associated with improved survival of patients with deeply infiltrating tumors. Int J Cancer 2011;128(2):379–89.
20. de Vos van Steenwijk PJ, Heusinkveld M, Ramwadhdoebe TH, et al. An unexpectedly large polyclonal repertoire of HPV-specific T cells is poised for action in patients with cervical cancer. Cancer Res 2010;70(7):2707–17.
21. Draper LM, Kwong ML, Gros A, et al. Targeting of HPV-16+ epithelial cancer cells by TCR gene engineered T cells directed against E6. Clin Cancer Res 2015; 21(19):4431–9.
22. Jin BY, Campbell TE, Draper LM, et al. Engineered T cells targeting E7 mediate regression of human papillomavirus cancers in a murine model. JCI Insight 2018;3(8):e99488..
23. Riemer AB, Keskin DB, Zhang G, et al. A conserved E7-derived cytotoxic T lymphocyte epitope expressed on human papillomavirus 16-transformed HLA-A2+ epithelial cancers. J Biol Chem 2010;285(38):29608–22.
24. Norberg S, Nagarsheth N, Sinkoe A,, et al. Safety and clinical activity of gene-engineered T-cell therapy targeting HPV-16 E7 for epithelial cancers. J Clin Oncol 2020;38(Suppl 15):101.
25. Ferris RL, Goncalves A, Baxi SS,, et al. An open-label, multicohort, phase 1/2 study in patients with virus-associated cancers (CheckMate 358): safety and efficacy of neoadjuvant nivolumab in squamous cell carcinoma of the head and neck (SCCHN). Ann Oncol 2017;28
26. Forde PM, Chaft JE, Smith KN,, et al. Neoadjuvant PD-1 blockade in resectable lung cancer. N Engl J Med 2018;378(21):1976–86.
27. Trinchieri G. Interleukin-12 and the regulation of innate resistance and adaptive immunity. Nat Rev Immunol 2003;3(2):133–46.
28. Weiss JM, Subleski JJ, Wigginton JM, et al. Immunotherapy of cancer by IL-12-based cytokine combinations. Expert Opin Biol Ther 2007;7(11):1705–21.
29. Leonard JP, Sherman ML, Fisher GL, et al. Effects of single-dose interleukin-12 exposure on interleukin-12-associated toxicity and interferon-gamma production. Blood 1997;90(7):2541–8.
30. Zhang L, Morgan RA, Beane JD,, et al. Tumor-infiltrating lymphocytes genetically engineered with an inducible gene encoding interleukin-12 for the immunotherapy of metastatic melanoma. Clin Cancer Res 2015;21(10):2278–88.
31. Zhang L, Davies JS, Serna C, et al. Enhanced efficacy and limited systemic cytokine exposure with membrane-anchored interleukin-12 T-cell therapy in murine tumor models. J Immunother Cancer 2020;8(1):e000210.
32. Rooney CM, Smith CA, Ng CY, et al. Use of gene-modified virus-specific T lymphocytes to control Epstein-Barr-virus-related lymphoproliferation. Lancet 1995; 345(8941):9–13.
33. Heslop HE, Slobod KS, Pule MA,, et al. Long-term outcome of EBV-specific T-cell infusions to prevent or treat EBV-related lymphoproliferative disease in transplant recipients. Blood 2010;115(5):925–35.
34. Zheng Y, Parsonage G, Zhuang X, et al. Human leukocyte antigen (HLA) A*1101-restricted Epstein-Barr virus-specific T-cell receptor gene transfer to target nasopharyngeal carcinoma. Cancer Immunol Res 2015;3(10):1138–47.
35. Caballero OL, Chen YT. Cancer/testis (CT) antigens: potential targets for immunotherapy. Cancer Sci 2009;100(11):2014–21.

36. Grossman RL, Heath AP, Ferretti V, et al. Toward a shared vision for cancer genomic data. N Engl J Med 2016;375(12):1109–12.
37. Kerkar SP, Wang ZF, Lasota J, et al. MAGE-A is more highly expressed than NY-ESO-1 in a systematic immunohistochemical analysis of 3668 cases. J Immunother 2016;39(4):181–7.
38. Shida A, Futawatari N, Fukuyama T, et al. Frequent high expression of Kita-Kyushu lung cancer antigen-1 (KK-LC-1) in gastric cancer. Anticancer Res 2015;35(6):3575–9.
39. Paret C, Simon P, Vormbrock K,, et al. CXorf61 is a target for T cell based immunotherapy of triple-negative breast cancer. Oncotarget 2015;6(28):25356–67.
40. Marcinkowski B, Stevanovic S, Helman SR,, et al. Cancer targeting by TCR gene-engineered T cells directed against Kita-Kyushu lung cancer antigen-1. J Immunother Cancer 2019;7(1):229.

Biologics for the Treatment of Recurrent Respiratory Papillomatosis

Clint T. Allen, MD

KEYWORDS

- Recurrent respiratory papillomatosis • Cidofovir • Bevacizumab • Immunotherapy

KEY POINTS

- Recurrent respiratory papillomatosis (RRP) is an infectious disorder resulting from the inability of the immune system to clear a chronic low-risk human papillomavirus infection.
- RRP is one of the few infectious disorders where repeat surgical intervention remains the standard of care.
- Adjuvant intralesional cidofovir remains widely used despite a paucity of prospective controlled data demonstrating clinical benefit.
- Antiangiogenic and immune activating adjuvant treatments may provide long-term clinical benefit based on known mechanisms of action for patients with RRP.

INTRODUCTION

Recurrent respiratory papillomatosis (RRP) is a neoplastic disorder that manifests as papillomatous growths in the upper aerodigestive tract. The symptom profile, socioeconomic implications, and standard treatment approaches have been outlined in recently published expert reviews.[1] Briefly, RRP, similar to anogenital condyloma, is caused by a chronic infection with low-risk human papillomavirus (HPV) types 6 or 11. Many are exposed to HPV 6 and 11, but few patients develop chronic infection and papillomatous disease. The genetic or environmental risk factors that dictate the development of a chronic infection or clearance of the low-risk HPV virus are poorly understood.[2] Diagnosis of papilloma by a trained pathologist is usually straightforward, and the recurrent nature and anatomic locations of disease point to the clinical diagnosis of RRP. Treatment of RRP has historically centered on maintenance surgical debulking of papillomatous disease aimed at providing the patient with a

Section on Translational Tumor Immunology, National Institute on Deafness and Other Communication Disorders, National Institutes of Health, Building 10, Room 7N240C, Bethesda, MD 20892, USA
E-mail address: Clint.allen@nih.gov

Otolaryngol Clin N Am 54 (2021) 769–777
https://doi.org/10.1016/j.otc.2021.05.002
0030-6665/21/Published by Elsevier Inc.

patent airway and a serviceable voice. RRP is one of the very few infectious disorders treated with repeat surgery.

Given the atypical clinical management of treating a chronic infectious disorder (as a result of presumed immune dysfunction) with repeat surgery not resulting in cure, adjuvant treatments used in combination with surgical debulking of disease or alternative treatments used in lieu of surgery have been studied. The inability or difficult nature of establishing in vitro or in vivo models of RRP has made research slow and challenging.[3,4] As a result, most published research in RRP is clinical research. Because large prospective clinical trials studying new RRP treatment are difficult to fund and accrue, most published clinical research studies are the result of small retrospective, uncontrolled, single-cohort studies. Many of these studies have contradictory results, leading to a lack of widespread acceptance of adjuvant treatments. Regardless, these efforts to establish to a biological treatment of RRP have focused on 3 main categories: the use of antivirals, antiangiogenics, or immunotherapy. Most reviews on adjuvant treatments for RRP have focused on antiviral or antiangiogenic therapy and mentioned immunotherapy in passing. Here, the authors do the opposite.

ANTIVIRAL THERAPY

Low-risk HPV is a DNA virus that encodes 8 proteins, and only one of these is an enzyme (E1). Thus, HPV relies on the host (infected cell) machinery for enzymes needed for replication, which is the primary reason why there are no antiviral drugs selective or specific for HPV—there are few HPV-specific proteins to attempt to inhibit.[5] Cidofovir is the antiviral drug most commonly used to treat active HPV infections. It was studied as an intralesional adjuvant following success as intralesional treatment of cytomegalovirus (CMV) retinitis.[6] The active metabolite of cidofovir, cidofovir diphosphate, selectively inhibits viral DNA polymerase and was specifically chosen for use in many other viral infections (such as CMV, where the virus encodes its own DNA polymerase) due to its ability to inhibit viral and not human DNA polymerase. Because HPV uses the host cell's DNA polymerase, the a priori expectation would be that cidofovir would require high concentrations to limit the replication of HPV. Cidofovir does seem to exert some antiproliferative effect on cells infected with HPV in culture, although the mechanisms of this inhibition are poorly understood.[7] Numerous groups have used locally injected cidofovir clinically (off-label, cidofovir is currently only Food and Drug Administration [FDA] approved for CMV retinitis) as an adjuvant treatment with surgical debulking of papillomatous disease, largely based on initial reports of clinical activity out of Europe in the 1990s.[8] Subsequent clinical reports have followed the pattern of many published on the topic of adjuvants in RRP—some studies show clinical benefit, whereas others do not. Ultimately a Cochrane review of the one prospective clinical trial to date on the use of cidofovir as an adjuvant for RRP treatment concluded no definitive evidence of clinical benefit.[9] Yet, given some positive retrospective studies on the use of intralesional cidofovir to prevent RRP recurrence, this adjuvant treatment is still used by select providers and institutions.

ANTIANGIOGENIC THERAPY

Because of the vascular nature of RRP lesions, biologics designed to disrupt blood vessel density or formation have been used clinically. Bevacizumab is a monoclonal antibody (mAb) that binds and prevents the activity of vascular endothelial growth factor (VEGF), thus destabilizing existing and preventing the formation of new blood vessels. The use of bevacizumab locally (intralesional injection) or systemically (intravenously) often results in profound regression of papillomatous disease in the upper aerodigestive tract,[10–15] presumably through blockade of papilloma blood supply. Several published clinical reports have been case series where systemic bevacizumab was used off-label (currently is FDA approved for multiple solid cancers) at different doses and schedules for patients with severe RRP. Use of bevacizumab for RRP has not been clinically studied prospectively, but anecdotally concerns over rebound papilloma growth with cessation of treatment have arisen. This concern has biological validity because VEGF blockade alone does not intrinsically activate HPV immunity. If the drug has to be stopped for whatever reason, the disease may regrow on withdrawal of the VEGF neutralization. Bevacizumab has a known side-effect profile (renal insufficiency),[16] and prospective studies are needed to determine optimum long-term dosing schedules aimed at keeping enough drug in the system to suppress papilloma growth while minimizing the risk of adverse events. The use of bevacizumab has garnered much attention based on dramatic examples of papillomatous disease regression while on drug in the literature, but significant questions surrounding duration of treatment and clinical plans on cessation of drug loom. These questions certainly deserve further study. Could bevacizumab be used clinically in combination with immunotherapy to both reduce the burden of disease and activate the immune system in the face of minimal residual disease? This approach seems to work well for highly vascular renal cell cancers.[17]

IMMUNOTHERAPY

Because RRP is a result of chronic infection, it can be thought of as an immune disorder. For some reason, the immune system of a patient with RRP does not clear the low-risk HPV infection. No specific immunodeficiencies resulting in increased risk of developing RRP have been identified, and patients with RRP in general are not immunocompromised. Whether this could be a problem with clearing HPV infections in general or whether this is a problem specific to low-risk HPV is unknown, but patients with RRP are not at higher risk of developing high-risk HPV infections.[18]

The T-lymphocyte (T cell) arm of the adaptive immune system is responsible for detecting and eliminating cells infected with a virus. Viral proteins produced inside infected epithelial cells are broken down (as all intracellular proteins), and small fragments of proteins called peptides are loaded onto major histocompatibility complex (MHC) class I molecules and moved to the surface of the cell. Here, T cells "sample" cells in passing, and when a T cell expresses a T-cell receptor that recognizes an MHC class I:peptide complex for which it is specific, the T cell kills the infected cell. The specific peptide that induced the response from the T cell is called a T-cell antigen. The more proteins a virus produces, the more of a chance that one or more peptides from those proteins can serve as a T-cell antigen; this has implications for low-risk HPVs that do not integrate into the host genome, remain episomal, and express most or all of their genes. Compared with high-risk HPVs that integrate E6 and E7 and tend to lose several or all other genes, low-risk HPVs produce a greater diversity of proteins, which may portend a greater chance of producing one or more T-cell antigens that would lead to the detection and elimination of infected cells; this may be one explanation for why fewer patients develop chronic low-risk HPV infections compared with the number of patients that develop chronic high-risk HPV infections.[19]

Several groups, particularly the Bonagura and Steinberg group out of Long Island Jewish, have firmly established the presence of local (within the papilloma) and systemic immunosuppression and T-cell dysfunction in patients with RRP. Papillomas from patients with RRP cells seem to have deficient (but seemingly rescuable) antigen processing and presentation of T-cell antigens,[20,21] and papillomas are full of immunosuppressive cells and cytokines that ultimately induce dysfunction in HPV-specific CD4 and CD8 T cells.[22–24] Clearly there are many mechanisms by which the papilloma microenvironment induces T-cell dysfunction, and this may contribute to the inability of T cells to detect and eliminate HPV-infected cells.

The Use of Immune Checkpoint Blockade to Unleash Existing Human Papillomavirus–Specific T Cells

Another mechanism by which HPV-infected epithelial cells could escape T-cell detection and elimination is the expression of immune checkpoints, the most popular of which are components of the programmed death (PD) pathway. When T cells are primed and activated (against, for example, an HPV antigen) they express the PD-1 inhibitory receptor. Activated T cells also produce interferon, which potently upregulates expression of the ligand for PD-1, PD-L1, on epithelial and stromal cells. This negative feedback loop to prevent uncontrolled T-cell activation results in suppression of T-cell activity. Therapeutic PD-1 or PD-L1 mAbs can disrupt this immune checkpoint axis and "unleash" the activity of existing T cells. Immune checkpoint blockade does not seem to induce new T-cell activity—it activates what already exists but is being suppressed by PD-1/L1 signaling. Indeed, T cells express PD-1, and PD-L1 expression is present on both papilloma cells and other infiltrating immune cells in most of the archived RRP samples.[25,26]

Our team reported the safety and clinical activity of PD-L1 blockade with avelumab in adult patients with aggressive RRP.[27] Most of the patients demonstrated significant reduction in papilloma disease burden without surgical debulking, and measurable amplification of HPV-specific T-cell responses was detected in several patients. At least one additional ongoing clinical trial of immune checkpoint blockade in RRP has reported similar results.[28] However, most of the patients were not cured with immune checkpoint blockade alone. Given that immune checkpoint blockade only activates existing T cells, this and other data suggested that inadequate T cell priming may be an issue in RRP. In other words, immunotherapy designed to activate new HPV-specific T-cell responses may be needed to eliminate HPV-infected cells and cure RRP.

The Use of Preventative Vaccines in the Therapeutic Setting

Understanding this framework of how virally infected cells are detected and eliminated by the T-cell arm of the adaptive immune system sets up one of the current clinical and scientific debates in this field of study. Preventative vaccines such as Gardasil induce a B lymphocyte (humoral) response that results in the production of antibodies.[29–31] HPV-specific antibodies can bind HPV virions, leading to their elimination by other arms of the immune system. There is no question this works, and prevention of HPV infection with Gardasil has already resulted in dramatically decreased incidence of RRP in Australia where vaccination is mandated.[32] Antibodies cannot, however, result in the detection and elimination of cells already infected with HPV. If the goal of the immunotherapy is to eliminate the cells already infected with HPV, only T cells can accomplish this task, and there is no evidence that preventative vaccines can educate or activate T cells. This biological understanding of how different arms of the adaptive immune system prevent or control existing infection is in conflict with clinical data suggesting that adjuvant administration of the Gardasil preventative vaccine prevents RRP disease recurrence or significantly lengthens the time between surgeries. Several single cohort, retrospective studies suggest a clinical benefit with increased intersurgery interval after adjuvant Gardasil administration.[29,33,34] Of 2 multicohort studies that reported intersurgery interval in patients with and without adjuvant Gardasil, one reported clinical benefit and the other did not.[35,36] Gardasil treatment does not increase the intersurgery interval in patients with low-risk HPV-associated anogenital condyloma.[37] The argument can be made that Gardasil is already commercially available, treatment is low risk, and that multiple HPV serotypes are covered that a patient may not have yet been exposed to, so patients with HPV-driven disorders should be treated regardless; this is clinically rational and may contribute to the most recent meta-analyses on the topic supporting the use of Gardasil as an adjuvant treatment in RRP despite the lack of convincing, prospective, controlled clinical data[38] and contrary conclusions being made in meta-analyses of data in other disease types driven by HPV.[39]

The Use of Therapeutic Vaccines in the Therapeutic Setting

Biologically rational, based on current understanding of immune responses against virally infected cells, is the design and clinical study of therapeutic vaccines for the treatment of established HPV infections. Such therapeutic vaccines come in many forms but share the goal of delivering HPV DNA to the innate immune cells (usually dendritic cells or macrophages) for T-cell priming and activation. *De novo* primed and activated HPV-specific T cells could then traffic to HPV-driven lesions and clear HPV-infected cells. The approach of using a therapeutic vaccine to induce strong T-cell responses and clinical benefit has already proved successful in the treatment of patients with premalignant cervical and vulvar intraepithelial neoplasia with a therapeutic vaccine encoding HPV 16 genes.[40,41]

Reports of clinical benefit with therapeutic vaccines for patients with RRP exist. In 2 trials, one using the MMR vaccine and the other using a modified vaccinia Ankara vector encoding the bovine papillomavirus E2 gene, intralesional injection of vaccine with or without surgical debulking of disease resulted in significant prolongation of the intersurgery interval or cure of disease in subsets of patients.[42,43] Neither report definitively demonstrated the induction of HPV-specific T-cell responses, suggesting that part or all of the clinical benefit induced with these treatments could be due to a local, nonspecific, antiviral inflammatory responses involving type I interferon (although such effects were not studied). More recently, report of clinical benefit in 3 patients treated with a DNA vaccine encoding HPV 6 E6 and E7 included demonstration of induction of HPV 6–specific T-cell responses.[44] These data have paved the path forward for multiple planned phase I and II clinical trials designed to study the safety and efficacy of novel therapeutic vaccines encoding HPV 6 and/or 11 genes.

SUMMARY

Clinical research is likely the path forward for the development of new monotherapy or adjuvant treatments for RRP, as the development of rapid and reproducible preclinical models has proved very difficult. There is no doubt that the use of bevacizumab locally or systemically is clinically active, but important fundamental questions such as dosing and duration of treatment need to be answered in prospective trials—for which funding is difficult to obtain. Advances will be made in the treatment of RRP, as treatments being clinically studied and ultimately FDA approved for HPV-associated cancers are translated into treatments for RRP; this is particularly true for immunotherapy, where the use of immune checkpoint blockade to activate preexisting HPV-specific T cells and therapeutic vaccines designed to generate new HPV-specific T-cell responses are now a reality. We now have the knowledge and tools needed to work, rationally and carefully, toward an immunologic cure of RRP.

CLINICS CARE POINTS

- Surgical debulking, as needed to maintain a patent airway and a serviceable voice, remains the standard of care treatment of RRP.
- Use of adjuvant intralesional cidofovir remains widespread despite a paucity of controlled prospective data demonstrating clinical benefit.
- Antiangiogenic targeted therapy with local or systemic bevacizumab can induce dramatic disease regression, but further study is required to assess the risk profile of long-term use.
- Immunotherapy in the form of immune checkpoint blockade or therapeutic vaccines may induce immune elimination of HPV-infected epithelial cells and hold promise for the control or cure of RRP.

FINANCIAL SUPPORT

This work was supported by the Intramural Research Program of the NIH, National Institute on Deafness and Other Communication Disorders, project number ZIA-DC00008.

ACKNOWLEDGMENTS

Thanks to Simon Best, MD (Johns Hopkins) and Pamela Mudd, MD (Children's National Hospital) for their critical review of this article.

DISCLOSURE

The author declares no conflicts of interest.

REFERENCES

1. Derkay CS, Bluher AE. Update on recurrent respiratory papillomatosis. Otolaryngol Clin North Am 2019;52(4):669–79.
2. Drutman SB, Haerynck F, Zhong FL, et al. Homozygous NLRP1 gain-of-function mutation in siblings with a syndromic form of recurrent respiratory papillomatosis. Proc Natl Acad Sci U S A 2019;116(38):19055–63.
3. Attra J, Hsieh LE, Luo L, et al. Development of human-derived cell culture lines for recurrent respiratory papillomatosis. Otolaryngol Head Neck Surg 2018;159(4):638–42.
4. Ahn J, Bishop JA, Akpeng B, et al. Xenograft model for therapeutic drug testing in recurrent respiratory papillomatosis. Ann Otol Rhinol Laryngol 2015;124(2):110–5.
5. Archambault J, Melendy T. Targeting human papillomavirus genome replication for antiviral drug discovery. Antivir Ther 2013;18(3):271–83.
6. Parenteral cidofovir for cytomegalovirus retinitis in patients with AIDS: the HPMPC peripheral cytomegalovirus retinitis trial. A randomized, controlled trial. Studies of Ocular complications of AIDS Research Group in Collaboration with the AIDS Clinical Trials Group. Ann Intern Med 1997;126(4):264–74.
7. Andrei G, Snoeck R, Piette J, et al. Antiproliferative effects of acyclic nucleoside phosphonates on human papillomavirus (HPV)-harboring cell lines compared with HPV-negative cell lines. Oncol Res 1998;10(10):523–31.

8. Van Cutsem E, Snoeck R, Van Ranst M, et al. Successful treatment of a squamous papilloma of the hypopharynx-esophagus by local injections of (S)-1-(3-hydroxy-2-phosphonylmethoxypropyl)cytosine. J Med Virol 1995;45(2):230–5.
9. Chadha NK, James A. Adjuvant antiviral therapy for recurrent respiratory papillomatosis. Cochrane Database Syst Rev 2012;12:CD005053.
10. Zeitels SM, Barbu AM, Landau-Zemer T, et al. Local injection of bevacizumab (Avastin) and angiolytic KTP laser treatment of recurrent respiratory papillomatosis of the vocal folds: a prospective study. Ann Otol Rhinol Laryngol 2011;120(10):627–34.
11. Hamdi O, Dome J, Zalzal G, et al. Systemic bevacizumab for end-stage juvenile recurrent respiratory papillomas: A case report. Int J Pediatr Otorhinolaryngol 2020;128:109706.
12. Bedoya A, Glisinski K, Clarke J, et al. Systemic bevacizumab for recurrent respiratory papillomatosis: a single center experience of two cases. Am J Case Rep 2017;18:842–6.
13. Best SR, Mohr M, Zur KB. Systemic bevacizumab for recurrent respiratory papillomatosis: a national survey. Laryngoscope 2017;127(10):2225–9.
14. Carnevale C, Ferran-De la Cierva L, Til-Perez G, et al. Safe use of systemic bevacizumab for respiratory recurrent papillomatosis in two children. Laryngoscope 2019;129(4):1001–4.
15. Mohr M, Schliemann C, Biermann C, et al. Rapid response to systemic bevacizumab therapy in recurrent respiratory papillomatosis. Oncol Lett 2014;8(5):1912–8.
16. Wu S, Kim C, Baer L, et al. Bevacizumab increases risk for severe proteinuria in cancer patients. J Am Soc Nephrol 2010;21(8):1381–9.
17. Dudek AZ, Liu LC, Gupta S, et al. Phase Ib/II clinical trial of pembrolizumab with bevacizumab for metastatic renal cell carcinoma: BTCRC-GU14-003. J Clin Oncol 2020;38(11):1138–45.
18. Omland T, Lie KA, Akre H, et al. Recurrent respiratory papillomatosis: HPV genotypes and risk of high-grade laryngeal neoplasia. PLoS One 2014;9(6):e99114.
19. Gillison ML, Alemany L, Snijders PJ, et al. Human papillomavirus and diseases of the upper airway: head and neck cancer and respiratory papillomatosis. Vaccine 2012;30(Suppl 5):F34–54.
20. Israr M, DeVoti JA, Lam F, et al. Altered monocyte and langerhans cell innate immunity in patients with recurrent respiratory papillomatosis (RRP). Front Immunol 2020;11:336.
21. Vambutas A, Bonagura VR, Reed EF, et al. Polymorphism of transporter associated with antigen presentation 1 as a potential determinant for severity of disease in recurrent respiratory papillomatosis caused by human papillomavirus types 6 and 11. J Infect Dis 2004;189(5):871–9.
22. Hatam LJ, Devoti JA, Rosenthal DW, et al. Immune suppression in premalignant respiratory papillomas: enriched functional CD4+Foxp3+ regulatory T cells and PD-1/PD-L1/L2 expression. Clin Cancer Res 2012;18(7):1925–35.
23. James EA, DeVoti JA, Rosenthal DW, et al. Papillomavirus-specific CD4+ T cells exhibit reduced STAT-5 signaling and altered cytokine profiles in patients with recurrent respiratory papillomatosis. J Immunol 2011;186(11):6633–40.
24. Bonagura VR, Vambutas A, DeVoti JA, et al. HLA alleles, IFN-gamma responses to HPV-11 E6, and disease severity in patients with recurrent respiratory papillomatosis. Hum Immunol 2004;65(8):773–82.
25. Ahn J, Bishop JA, Roden RBS, et al. The PD-1 and PD-L1 pathway in recurrent respiratory papillomatosis. Laryngoscope 2018;128(1):E27–32.

26. Liu T, Greenberg M, Wentland C, et al. PD-L1 expression and CD8+ infiltration shows heterogeneity in juvenile recurrent respiratory papillomatosis. Int J Pediatr Otorhinolaryngol 2017;95:133–8.
27. Allen CT, Lee S, Norberg SM, et al. Safety and clinical activity of PD-L1 blockade in patients with aggressive recurrent respiratory papillomatosis. J Immunother Cancer 2019;7(1):119.
28. Pai SI, Friedman AD, Franco R, et al. A phase II study of pembrolizumab for HPV-associated papilloma patients with laryngeal, tracheal, and/or pulmonary involvement. J Clin Oncol 2019;37(15_suppl):2502.
29. Tjon Pian Gi RE, San Giorgi MR, Pawlita M, et al. Immunological response to quadrivalent HPV vaccine in treatment of recurrent respiratory papillomatosis. Eur Arch Otorhinolaryngol 2016;273(10):3231–6.
30. Li L, Zhang Z, Fu C. The subjective well-being effect of public goods provided by village collectives: evidence from China. PLoS One 2020;15(3):e0230065.
31. Zhang CQ, Yi S, Liu XJ, et al. Safety and immunogenicity of a nonadjuvant human papillomavirus type 6 virus-like particle vaccine in recurrent respiratory papillomatosis. J Voice 2019;33(3):363–9.
32. Novakovic D, Cheng ATL, Zurynski Y, et al. A prospective study of the incidence of juvenile-onset recurrent respiratory papillomatosis after implementation of a National HPV Vaccination Program. J Infect Dis 2018;217(2):208–12.
33. Young DL, Moore MM, Halstead LA. The use of the quadrivalent human papillomavirus vaccine (gardasil) as adjuvant therapy in the treatment of recurrent respiratory papilloma. J Voice 2015;29(2):223–9.
34. Matsuzaki H, Makiyama K, Hirai R, et al. Multi-year effect of human papillomavirus vaccination on recurrent respiratory papillomatosis. Laryngoscope 2020;130(2):442–7.
35. Milner TD, Harrison A, Montgomery J, et al. A retrospective case-control analysis of the efficacy of Gardasil((R)) vaccination in 28 patients with recurrent respiratory papillomatosis of the larynx. Clin Otolaryngol 2018;43(3):962–5.
36. Mauz PS, Schafer FA, Iftner T, et al. HPV vaccination as preventive approach for recurrent respiratory papillomatosis - a 22-year retrospective clinical analysis. BMC Infect Dis 2018;18(1):343.
37. Husein-ElAhmed H. Could the human papillomavirus vaccine prevent recurrence of ano-genital warts?: a systematic review and meta-analysis. Int J STD AIDS 2020;31(7):606–12.
38. Rosenberg T, Philipsen BB, Mehlum CS, et al. Therapeutic use of the human papillomavirus vaccine on recurrent respiratory papillomatosis: a systematic review and meta-analysis. J Infect Dis 2019;219(7):1016–25.
39. Hampl M, Sarajuuri H, Wentzensen N, et al. Effect of human papillomavirus vaccines on vulvar, vaginal, and anal intraepithelial lesions and vulvar cancer. Obstet Gynecol 2006;108(6):1361–8.
40. Kenter GG, Welters MJ, Valentijn AR, et al. Vaccination against HPV-16 oncoproteins for vulvar intraepithelial neoplasia. N Engl J Med 2009;361(19):1838–47.
41. van Poelgeest MI, Welters MJ, Vermeij R, et al. Vaccination against Oncoproteins of HPV16 for noninvasive vulvar/vaginal lesions: lesion clearance is related to the strength of the T-cell response. Clin Cancer Res 2016;22(10):2342–50.
42. Wang Y, Dai PD, Zhang TY. Experimental research on the therapeutic effect of MMR vaccine to juvenile-onset recurrent respiratory papillomatosis. Eur Arch Otorhinolaryngol 2019;276(3):801–3.

43. Cabo Beltran OR, Rosales Ledezma R. MVA E2 therapeutic vaccine for marked reduction in likelihood of recurrence of respiratory papillomatosis. Head Neck 2019;41(3):657–65.
44. Aggarwal C, Cohen RB, Morrow MP, et al. Immune therapy targeting E6/E7 oncogenes of human paillomavirus type 6 (HPV-6) reduces or eliminates the need for surgical intervention in the treatment of HPV-6 associated recurrent respiratory papillomatosis. Vaccines (Basel) 2020;8(1):56.

Past and Future Biologics for Otologic Disorders

Steven A. Gordon, MD, MPH, Richard K. Gurgel, MD, MSCI*

KEYWORDS

- Biologics • Gene therapy • Growth factors • Tympanic membrane regeneration
- Hearing preservation

KEY POINTS

- Although none of the novel products under investigation has yet made it to the clinical market, many therapeutics have entered clinical testing and more are expected to do so in the next few years.
- Growth factors, such as insulinlike growth factor and basic fibroblast growth factor, have shown promising results with hearing preservation and tympanic membrane regeneration, respectively.
- Apoptosis inhibitors, such as AM-111, demonstrated promising results for treatment of idiopathic sudden sensorineural loss as salvage therapy.
- The first trial of gene therapy for the treatment of deafness in humans was in March 2020.

INTRODUCTION

Hearing loss is the most common sensory deficit in the general population, with approximately 500 million people afflicted.[1] Among those patients, approximately 90% have a diagnosis of sensorineural loss.[2] Despite an increasing age of the population with an increasing incidence of hearing loss, there are no approved pharmacologic or biological therapies targeting this problem. Currently, the only option for patients in whom hearing loss cannot be rehabilitated with hearing aids is through cochlear implantation (CI).[3] Although CIs offer the ability to hear for individuals with severe to profound sensorineural hearing loss, they are inherently limited in their ability to restore "natural" hearing. To combat this limitation, researchers and scientists have sought to study and develop new technologies in regenerating the inner ear. To date, a total of 43 biotechnology and pharmaceutical therapeutics for inner ear and central hearing disorders are under investigation.[1] These therapeutics include drug-based, cell-based, and gene-based approaches to prevent hearing loss or its

Otolaryngology–Head & Neck Surgery, University of Utah Health, 50 North Medical Drive 3C120 SOM, Salt Lake City, UT 84132, USA
* Corresponding author.
E-mail address: Richard.Gurgel@hsc.utah.edu

Otolaryngol Clin N Am 54 (2021) 779–787
https://doi.org/10.1016/j.otc.2021.05.003
0030-6665/21/Published by Elsevier Inc.

progression, restore hearing, and regenerate the inner ear (**Fig. 1**). Although none of the novel products under investigation has yet made it to the clinical market,[1] many therapeutics have entered clinical testing and more are expected to do so in the next few years.

Because these developing therapies have the ability to change the management of hearing loss fundamentally, clinicians need to familiarize themselves with their prospective application in practice. This article reviews the current application of 4 categories of biological therapeutics—growth factors, apoptosis inhibitors, monoclonal antibodies, and gene therapy—in otology and their potential future directions and applications.

GROWTH FACTORS

Insulinlike Growth Factor 1

Biological therapy to treat inner ear pathology still is a nascent science. Activation of numerous cellular signaling pathways has the potential to trigger both protective and regenerative outcomes in the central nervous system. Based on a multitude of emerging and investigative studies, numerous therapeutics have been recognized as protective in the inner ear. For instance, the administration of different growth factors has exhibited both preservation of spiral ganglion neurons and regeneration of neuritic processes.[4–6] One promising substance is insulinlike growth factor 1 (IGF-1) because it plays a vital role for inner ear development.[7] Within the central nervous system, IGF-1 and its receptor regulate neuronal survival, differentiation, and neurogenesis.[8] IGF-1 injection at the round window has been studied in rats and guinea pigs with noise-induced hearing loss and found to have a protective benefit.[7,9] Similarly, in a different guinea pig model, IGF-1 administration improved hearing preservation at lower frequencies, 7 days after CI.[10] In the IGF-1–treated group, histologic studies revealed that outer hair cell numbers were maintained in the cochlear region

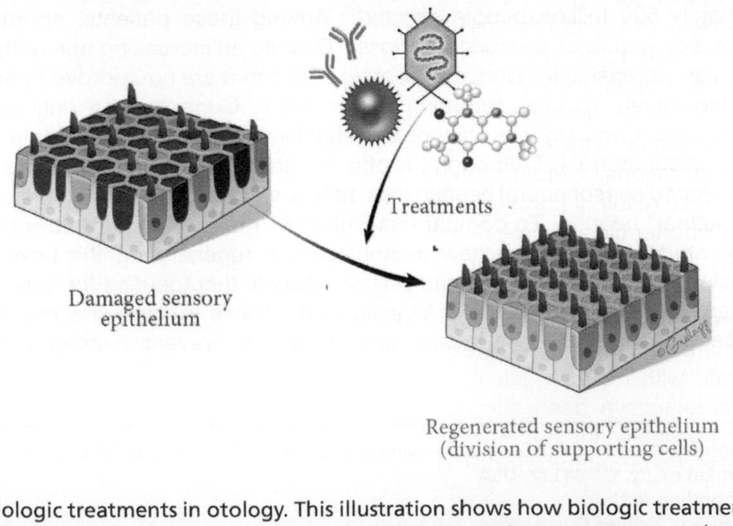

Fig. 1. Biologic treatments in otology. This illustration shows how biologic treatments could be used in otology to regenerate or repair the inner ear. Various treatments, such as growth factors, apoptosis inhibitors, monoclonal antibodies, and gene therapy via viral vectors, could be used in the future to treat disorders of the inner ear. (*Courtesy of* Chris Gralapp, Christine Gralapp Medical Illustration, Fairfax, CA; printed with permission © Chris Gralapp.)

responsible for low-frequency hearing (upper basal to midbasal turn) and that there was less fibrous tissue formation around the electrode.[10]

Additionally, IGF-1 has been applied in a phase 1 study by a group in Japan in 26 patients who failed steroid therapy for idiopathic sudden sensorineural hearing loss (ISSHL). These researchers applied gelatin hydrogels, impregnated with recombinant human IGF-1 into the middle ear adjacent to the round window niche during tympanostomy under local anesthesia. Subjects then were hospitalized for 4 days postoperatively. In comparison to a historical control of ISSHL patients treated with hyperbaric oxygen, in which 33% of patients showed pure tone threshold improvement 12 weeks after treatment, 48% of the IGF-1 group showed improvement ($P = .08$).[11] There were no adverse events reported with IGF-1 administration.

Although still in early development, animal investigations analyzing topical IGF-1's efficacy for facial nerve regeneration have shown positive results. One group studied guinea pigs that were treated with either IGF-1 or saline, which was administered topically by a gelatin-based sustained-release hydrogel via an intratemporal route.[12] The recovery from facial nerve palsy was evaluated at 8 weeks postoperatively based on eyelid closure, complete recovery rate, electroneurography, and number of axons found on the facial nerve. IGF-1 treatment resulted in significant improvement in the changes of the degree of eyelid closure over the total time period and complete recovery rate.[12] Similar results were found in a rabbit model following crush injury to the facial nerve. In the IGF-1–treated group, axonal order and myelin were reportedly preserved, and Schwann cell proliferation was close to normal compared with a control group ($P<.05$).[13]

Basic Fibroblast Growth Factor and Epidermal Growth Factor

Other growth factors, such as epidermal growth factor (EGF) and basic fibroblast growth factor (bFGF), have been studied to treat otologic disorders. With advancements in the field of tissue engineering, various bioscaffolds have been impregnated with these growth factors with encouraging results for tympanic membrane (TM) repair. To date, there have been 14 studies evaluating bFGF with a control group in the humans, 7 of which are considered randomized controlled trials between 2003 and 2018.[14] A meta-analysis of these studies demonstrated closure rates for acute perforations treated with growth factors to range from 89% to 100% (median 97.5%) in the bFGF groups and 53% to 90% (median 79.5%) in the control groups ($P<.01$).[14] A similar statistically significant result was seen in 2 studies examining chronic perforations.[14] Most of these studies examined posttraumatic perforations that were not a result of chronic infection. The studies additionally found a statistically significant shorter closing time of these perforations in 524 participants in 7 studies.[14] Ultimately, there was no difference in hearing outcomes compared with their controls.[14] There have been 2 human trials comprising 215 patients treated with EGF-impregnated bioscaffolds for traumatic TM perforation. One study found no improvement for chronic perforations, whereas another described near-complete closure rate with EGF on gelatin sponge for acute perforations.[15,16] Both of these growth factors have been shown effective in minimally invasive procedures with limited to no significant side effects.[17] The EGF receptor also has been shown as a novel molecular target for aggressive papillary tumors in the middle ear and temporal bone.[18]

Platelet-Derived Growth Factor/Platelet-Rich Plasma/Hyaluronic Acid

The application of platelet-derived growth factor (PDGF) in acute TM perforations in rats was found to heal several days quicker than controls.[19] Histologic examination revealed a more substantial fibrous connective tissue layer in the PDGF-treated TMs, suggesting that a more physiologic trilaminar TM could be generated using this growth factor. No adverse events were observed.[19] A more recent study, however, analyzed topical application of PDGF as an office treatment of TM perforation as a result of chronic otitis media versus placebo and found no improvement in closure rate because most patients ultimately required surgical repair in both groups.[20]

One study has analyzed acute TM perforation in 20 rats who were treated with autologous platelet-rich plasma (PRP) in 1 ear and using the anima'ls other ear as a control.[21] The mean healing time for the PRP-treated TM was significantly shorter than the control TM. On histopathologic examination, however, no significant differences were noted between the 2 groups.

A similar investigation into the effectiveness of hyaluronic acid (HA), and its commercially available esterfied form, MeroGel (Medtronic Xomed, Jacksonville, Florida), was performed in 24 rats randomized into (1) single application of MeroGel to right TM and (2) daily application of topical 1% HA to right TM. The left TMs served as controls.[22] On the seventh day, the following closure rates were observed: MeroGel, 91.7%; topical HA, 100%; and control, 70.85%. Both study groups had significantly greater closure rates than the control group (no difference was noted between the study groups).[22] The investigators favored the use of MeroGel due to its single application regimen.

Vascular Endothelial Growth Factor

Vascular endothelial growth factor (VEGF) has many applications in the ear.[23] The expression of VEGF has been reported in the middle ear in response to inflammatory stimuli. VEGF expression was identified in effusion fluid and middle ear mucosa of human patients with otitis media.[24] One study treated mice once daily with 3 different VEGF receptor inhibitors. Hearing was assessed from day 28 to day 56, and all 3 of these inhibitors significantly decreased hearing loss.[25] Clinical trials using systemic anti-VEGF treatment have inherent limitations due to the side-effect profile of anti-VEGF treatment, which includes delayed wound healing, hemorrhage, and thrombosis. These potential side effects may not be acceptable in the treatment of a non–life-threatening disease, such as otitis media with effusion.[26] Anti-VEGF therapy via the transtympanic route may be a viable treatment option that minimizes systemic side effects.[25]

APOPTOSIS INHIBITORS

More recent studies have begun investigating alterations in the pathway of apoptosis as a treatment strategy for hearing protection. Studies evaluating AM-111, a c-Jun N-terminal kinase (JNK) inhibitor, have determined positive protective effect against noise-induced trauma.[27] These findings suggest that AM-111 plays a key role in mediating cochlear sensory cell death from oxidative stress. Similar conclusions were observed in an animal model in which the application of AM-111 helped safeguard against hair cell loss following labyrinthitis. This compound was determined to be successful in preventing hearing loss from electrode insertion trauma in a guinea pig model.[28] Treatment with AM-111 prevented the progressive worsening of auditory brainstem response (ABR) thresholds and decrease in distortion product otoacoustic emissions amplitudes that occur after electrode insertion trauma in the study guinea pigs.[28] When AM-111 was analyzed in its ability to protect against cisplatin-induced hearing loss, it was not effective.[29] Its use recently has undergone a phase II clinical trial for treatment of ISSNHL as salvage therapy. In this investigation, significant benefits of JNK inhibitors were seen in subjects with severe hearing loss 30 days after onset of symptoms. Specifically, in severe to profound ISSNHL patients (threshold $\geq$60 dB), JNK inhibitors showed statistically significant, clinically relevant, and persistent improvements in hearing and speech discrimination and higher tinnitus remission compared with placebo.[30] In contrast, JNK inhibitor treatment provided after 90 days of symptom onset, saw limited to no effect.[30]

MONOCLONAL ANTIBODY

Monoclonal antibody therapy is incorporated most commonly in the treatment of autoimmune inner ear disease causing progressive hearing loss and is described in detail in another article. However, 1 preliminary study has shown inner ear protective effect of etanercept, a tumor necrosis factor (TNF) inhibitor that fuses the TNF receptor to the end of an IgG1 antibody. When etanercept was delivered via an osmotic minipump into the scala tympani, it improved hearing preservation rates during CI insertion in guinea pigs.[31]

GENE THERAPY

The simple and prevailing objective of gene transfer technology is to introduce a therapeutic gene, for example, a normal version of the defective gene, into appropriate target cells of the affected individual. Expression of the exogenous therapeutic gene then would alter the target cell and the clinical phenotype. The integration of gene therapy for ear-related conditions generally has targeted genetic disorders, hair cell regeneration, and delivery of neurotrophins to the inner ear.[32] Although gene delivery is invasive, clinical trials currently are under way to evaluate its safety and efficacy in the preservation and regeneration of inner and outer hair cells.

Gene therapy treatment success is largely dictated by the success on the gene delivery system, often termed, the *vector*. This vector is implanted with the goal of transferring the gene to identified target cells, with a persistent and effective expression of the transgene in target cells. Currently, the most promising delivery system for gene therapy is through the use of viral vectors. At least 5 types of viral vectors used for gene therapy have been examined: retroviruses, lentiviruses,[33–36] adenoviruses, and adeno-associated viruses (AAVs),[37–42] and herpes simplex virus.[43,44]

The most encouraging results have been demonstrated using AAVs in animal studies. In the inner ear, AAV1-4, AAV1-7, and AAV1-8 have been shown to transduce spiral ligament, spiral limbus, and spiral ganglion cells. AAV-5 also was shown to be efficient for transducing Claudius cells, sulcus cells, and spiral ganglion neurons.[39,45–49] Similarly, AAV1-3, AAV1-5, AAV1-6, and AAV1-8 transduce IHCs. AAV-1 is the most effective transducer of outer hair cells and supporting cells.[50,51]

Initial inner ear gene therapy trials using AAVs as viral vectors with the basic helix-loop-helix transcription factor protein atonal homolog 1 (Atoh1), also known as MATH1, has shown that this transcription factor is required for the differentiation of hair cells.[52] In animal studies, gene therapy with delivery of MATH1 has been shown to induce hair cell regeneration.[53,54] Encouraging results have been obtained in vitro and in animals, particularly by overexpressing the Math1 transcription factor, which is both necessary and sufficient to induce the differentiation of hair cells in the mammalian cochlea. Guinea pigs rendered deaf by exposure to ototoxic drugs given an AAV carrying the Math1 gene triggered the formation of new auditory hair cells through the trans differentiation of support cells.[55] In March 2020, the first trial of gene therapy for the treatment of deafness in humans was launched in the United States by a team led by Dr Hinrich Staecker.[56] Their objective is to deliver a Math1-

expressing adenovirus to the cochlea of these patients with severe to profound sensorineural hearing loss, with the aim of evaluating the safety of the treatment.

FUTURE DIRECTIONS

The development of stem cell therapies for the inner ear opens a range of therapeutic possibilities. Initially, cells could be developed to deliver growth factors or even as a vehicle for gene therapy. In pilot studies, lentivirus-modified cells survived for 21 days in the guinea pig cochlea.[33] This would allow the delivery of neurotrophins at a high concentration for 3 weeks without the need for a pump or viral vector. Additional growth factors produced by these cells could mitigate inflammatory reactions induced by CI and improve hearing preservation. Potentially, cell therapy could be used to replace existing cells with a genetic defect.

SUMMARY

The effective implementation of biologic therapy has the ability to redefine how to prevent hearing loss or its progression, restore hearing, and regenerate the inner ear. As described, the most promising means of study include drug-based, cell-based and gene-based approaches (a visual representation is in **Fig. 1**). Therapeutics, such as IGF-1, AM-111, and etanercept, offer potential to protect against fibrosis and maintain auditory cells in hearing preservation CI. Growth factors EGF, bFGF, platelet-derived growth factor, PRP, and HA have been shown effective for TM regeneration in traumatic perforations with the possibility of further benefit for chronic infectious disease. Moreover, adenoviral-mediated MATH1 gene delivery has shown promising results in vivo for regenerating inner ear hair cells and currently is under phase 1/2 clinical trial. The vast diversity of therapeutics under development is a direct reflection of the intricacies of the inner ear and central hearing disorders as well as the complexity of this research. To better care for the growing number of patients suffering from hearing loss, it is imperative for providers to prepare and educate themselves on the potential therapeutics available and be ready to incorporate them into their practice when suitable.

CLINICS CARE POINTS

- IGF-1 plays a vital role for inner ear development. Its administration in a guinea pig model demonstrated improved hearing preservation at lower frequencies, 7 days after CI.
- bFGF and EGF growth factors have been shown effective in minimally invasive procedures to close traumatic perforations with limited to no significant side effects.
- Specifically, in severe to profound ISSNHL patients (threshold $\geq$60 dB), JNK inhibitors showed statistically significant, clinically relevant, and persistent improvements in hearing and speech discrimination and higher tinnitus remission compared with placebo in a phase II trial.

DISCLOSURE

Sources of financial support or funding: none. Declarations of interest: none.

REFERENCES

1. Schilder AGM, Su MP, Blackshaw H, et al. Hearing protection, restoration, and regeneration: an overview of emerging therapeutics for inner ear and central hearing disorders. Otol Neurotol 2019;40:559–70.

2. Patel NP, Mhatre AN, Lalwani AK. Biological therapy for the inner ear. Expert Opin Biol Ther 2004;4:1811–9.
3. Buchman CA, Gifford RH, Haynes DS, et al. Unilateral cochlear implants for severe, profound, or moderate sloping to profound bilateral sensorineural hearing loss: a systematic review and consensus statements. JAMA Otolaryngol Head Neck Surg 2020;146(10):942–53.
4. Shibata SB, Budenz CL, Bowling SA, et al. Nerve maintenance and regeneration in the damaged cochlea. Hear Res 2011;281:56–64.
5. Wise AK, Gillespie LN. Drug delivery to the inner ear. J Neural Eng 2012;9:065002.
6. Yamamoto N, Nakagawa T, Ito J. Application of insulin-like growth factor-1 in the treatment of inner ear disorders. Front Pharmacol 2014;5:208.
7. Lee KY, Nakagawa T, Okano T, et al. Novel therapy for hearing loss: delivery of insulin-like growth factor 1 to the cochlea using gelatin hydrogel. Otol Neurotol 2007;28:976–81.
8. Digicaylioglu M, Garden G, Timberlake S, et al. Acute neuroprotective synergy of erythropoietin and insulin-like growth factor I. Proc Natl Acad Sci U S A 2004;101:9855–60.
9. Iwai K, Nakagawa T, Endo T, et al. Cochlear protection by local insulin-like growth factor-1 application using biodegradable hydrogel. Laryngoscope 2006;116:529–33.
10. Yamahara K, Nishimura K, Ogita H, et al. Hearing preservation at low frequencies by insulin-like growth factor 1 in a guinea pig model of cochlear implantation. Hear Res 2018;368:92–108.
11. Nakagawa T, Sakamoto T, Hiraumi H, et al. Topical insulin-like growth factor 1 treatment using gelatin hydrogels for glucocorticoid-resistant sudden sensorineural hearing loss: a prospective clinical trial. BMC Med 2010;8:76.
12. Sugiyama M, Ito T, Furukawa T, et al. The effect of insulin-like growth factor 1 on the recovery of facial nerve function in a guinea pig model of facial palsy. J Physiol Sci 2020;70:28.
13. Bayrak AF, Olgun Y, Ozbakan A, et al. The effect of insulin like growth factor-1 on recovery of facial nerve crush injury. Clin Exp Otorhinolaryngol 2017;10:296–302.
14. Huang J, Teh BM, Eikelboom RH, et al. The effectiveness of bfgf in the treatment of tympanic membrane perforations: a systematic review and meta-analysis. Otol Neurotol 2020;41:782–90.
15. Lou ZC, Dong Y, Lou ZH. Comparative study of epidermal growth factor and observation only on human subacute tympanic membrane perforation. Am J Otolaryngol 2019;40:209–12.
16. Ramsay HA, Heikkonen EJ, Laurila PK. Effect of epidermal growth factor on tympanic membranes with chronic perforations: a clinical trial. Otolaryngol Head Neck Surg 1995;113:375–9.
17. Acharya AN, Coates H, Tavora-Vieira D, et al. A pilot study investigating basic fibroblast growth factor for the repair of chronic tympanic membrane perforations in pediatric patients. Int J Pediatr Otorhinolaryngol 2015;79:332–5.
18. Kawabata S, Hollander MC, Munasinghe JP, et al. Epidermal growth factor receptor as a novel molecular target for aggressive papillary tumors in the middle ear and temporal bone. Oncotarget 2015;6:11357–68.
19. Yeo SW, Kim SW, Suh BD, et al. Effects of platelet-derived growth factor-AA on the healing process of tympanic membrane perforation. Am J Otolaryngol 2000;21:153–60.

20. Roosli C, von Buren T, Gassmann NB, et al. The impact of platelet-derived growth factor on closure of chronic tympanic membrane perforations: a randomized, double-blind, placebo-controlled study. Otol Neurotol 2011;32:1224–9.
21. Erkilet E, Koyuncu M, Atmaca S, et al. Platelet-rich plasma improves healing of tympanic membrane perforations: experimental study. J Laryngol Otol 2009; 123:482–7.
22. Ozturk K, Yaman H, Cihat Avunduk M, et al. Effectiveness of MeroGel hyaluronic acid on tympanic membrane perforations. Acta Otolaryngol 2006;126:1158–63.
23. London NR, Gurgel RK. The role of vascular endothelial growth factor and vascular stability in diseases of the ear. Laryngoscope 2014;124:E340–6.
24. Jung HH, Kim MW, Lee JH, et al. Expression of vascular endothelial growth factor in otitis media. Acta Otolaryngol 1999;119:801–8.
25. Cheeseman MT, Tyrer HE, Williams D, et al. HIF-VEGF pathways are critical for chronic otitis media in Junbo and Jeff mouse mutants. Plos Genet 2011;7: e1002336.
26. Kamba T, McDonald DM. Mechanisms of adverse effects of anti-VEGF therapy for cancer. Br J Cancer 2007;96:1788–95.
27. Coleman JK, Littlesunday C, Jackson R, et al. AM-111 protects against permanent hearing loss from impulse noise trauma. Hear Res 2007;226:70–8.
28. Eshraghi AA, He J, Mou CH, et al. D-JNKI-1 treatment prevents the progression of hearing loss in a model of cochlear implantation trauma. Otol Neurotol 2006;27: 504–11.
29. Wang J, Ladrech S, Pujol R, et al. Caspase inhibitors, but not c-Jun NH2-terminal kinase inhibitor treatment, prevent cisplatin-induced hearing loss. Cancer Res 2004;64:9217–24.
30. Suckfuell M, Lisowska G, Domka W, et al. Efficacy and safety of AM-111 in the treatment of acute sensorineural hearing loss: a double-blind, randomized, placebo-controlled phase II study. Otol Neurotol 2014;35:1317–26.
31. Ihler F, Pelz S, Coors M, et al. Application of a TNF-alpha-inhibitor into the scala tympany after cochlear electrode insertion trauma in guinea pigs: preliminary audiologic results. Int J Audiol 2014;53:810–6.
32. Roemer A, Staecker H, Sasse S, et al. Biological therapies in otology. HNO 2017; 65:87–97.
33. Han JJ, Mhatre AN, Wareing M, et al. Transgene expression in the guinea pig cochlea mediated by a lentivirus-derived gene transfer vector. Hum Gene Ther 1999;10:1867–73.
34. Pietola L, Aarnisalo AA, Joensuu J, et al. HOX-GFP and WOX-GFP lentivirus vectors for inner ear gene transfer. Acta Otolaryngol 2008;128:613–20.
35. Wei Y, Fu Y, Liu S, et al. Effect of lentiviruses carrying enhanced green fluorescent protein injected into the scala media through a cochleostomy in rats. Am J Otolaryngol 2013;34:301–7.
36. Wang Y, Sun Y, Chang Q, et al. Early postnatal virus inoculation into the scala media achieved extensive expression of exogenous green fluorescent protein in the inner ear and preserved auditory brainstem response thresholds. J Gene Med 2013;15:123–33.
37. Suzuki M, Yamasoba T, Suzukawa K, et al. Adenoviral vector gene delivery via the round window membrane in guinea pigs. Neuroreport 2003;14:1951–5.
38. Yang J, Cong N, Han Z, et al. Ectopic hair cell-like cell induction by Math1 mainly involves direct transdifferentiation in neonatal mammalian cochlea. Neurosci Lett 2013;549:7–11.

39. Chien WW, Monzack EL, McDougald DS, et al. Gene therapy for sensorineural hearing loss. Ear Hear 2015;36:1–7.
40. Husseman J, Raphael Y. Gene therapy in the inner ear using adenovirus vectors. Adv Otorhinolaryngol 2009;66:37–51.
41. Sacheli R, Delacroix L, Vandenackerveken P, et al. Gene transfer in inner ear cells: a challenging race. Gene Ther 2013;20:237–47.
42. Naso MF, Tomkowicz B, Perry WL 3rd, et al. Adeno-Associated Virus (AAV) as a Vector for Gene Therapy. BioDrugs 2017;31:317–34.
43. Chen X, Frisina RD, Bowers WJ, et al. HSV amplicon-mediated neurotrophin-3 expression protects murine spiral ganglion neurons from cisplatin-induced damage. Mol Ther 2001;3:958–63.
44. Derby ML, Sena-Esteves M, Breakefield XO, et al. Gene transfer into the mammalian inner ear using HSV-1 and vaccinia virus vectors. Hear Res 1999;134:1–8.
45. Kilpatrick LA, Li Q, Yang J, et al. Adeno-associated virus-mediated gene delivery into the scala media of the normal and deafened adult mouse ear. Gene Ther 2011;18:569–78.
46. Chien WW, McDougald DS, Roy S, et al. Cochlear gene transfer mediated by adeno-associated virus: Comparison of two surgical approaches. Laryngoscope 2015;125:2557–64.
47. Li Duan M, Bordet T, Mezzina M, et al. Adenoviral and adeno-associated viral vector mediated gene transfer in the guinea pig cochlea. Neuroreport 2002;13: 1295–9.
48. Liu Y, Okada T, Sheykholeslami K, et al. Specific and efficient transduction of Cochlear inner hair cells with recombinant adeno-associated virus type 3 vector. Mol Ther 2005;12:725–33.
49. Ballana E, Wang J, Venail F, et al. Efficient and specific transduction of cochlear supporting cells by adeno-associated virus serotype 5. Neurosci Lett 2008;442: 134–9.
50. Akil O, Seal RP, Burke K, et al. Restoration of hearing in the VGLUT3 knockout mouse using virally mediated gene therapy. Neuron 2012;75:283–93.
51. Askew C, Rochat C, Pan B, et al. Tmc gene therapy restores auditory function in deaf mice. Sci Transl Med 2015;7:295ra108.
52. Bermingham NA, Hassan BA, Price SD, et al. Math1: an essential gene for the generation of inner ear hair cells. Science 1999;284:1837–41.
53. Staecker H, Praetorius M, Baker K, et al. Vestibular hair cell regeneration and restoration of balance function induced by math1 gene transfer. Otol Neurotol 2007;28:223–31.
54. Izumikawa M, Minoda R, Kawamoto K, et al. Auditory hair cell replacement and hearing improvement by Atoh1 gene therapy in deaf mammals. Nat Med 2005; 11:271–6.
55. Kawamoto K, Ishimoto S, Minoda R, et al. Math1 gene transfer generates new cochlear hair cells in mature guinea pigs in vivo. J Neurosci 2003;23:4395–400.
56. Safety, Tolerability and Efficacy for CGF166 in Patients With Unilateral or Bilateral Severe-to-profound Hearing Loss [type]. ClinicalTrials.gov; 2020.

Biological Treatments of Neurofibromatosis Type 2 and Other Skull Base Disorders

Scott Raskin, DO[a,b], Miriam Bornhorst, MD[a,b,c,*]

KEYWORDS

- Biological therapy • Neurofibromatosis type 2 • von Hippel–Lindau • Chordoma
- Meningioma • Vestibular schwannoma • Paraganglioma • Endolymphatic sac tumor

KEY POINTS

- Treatment of skull base tumors, including tumors associated with neurofibromatosis type 2 and other cancer predisposition syndromes, is a multidisciplinary approach.
- Molecularly targeted therapies, including vascular endothelial growth factor inhibitors, tyrosine kinase inhibitors, and mammalian target of rapamycin complex inhibitors, show promise in clinical trials for many skull base tumors.
- Future studies should focus on novel combination biological therapies to further advance treatment options in patients with skull base tumors.

INTRODUCTION

Skull base tumors are rare tumors that grow either within the cranial base or between the brain and base of the skull.[1] They include tumors, such as schwannomas (vestibular schwannomas [VSs]), meningiomas, chordomas, chondrosarcomas, endolymphatic sac tumors (ELSTs), craniopharyngiomas, carcinomas, neuroblastomas, and paragangliomas. With the exception of some neuroblastomas, sarcomas, and carcinomas, many skull base tumors do not respond well to chemotherapy and have been treated primarily with surgery with or without radiation therapy (RT).[2,3] Both surgery and RT carry major potential risk to nearby structures as well as possibility of tumor transformation, especially for neurofibromatosis type 2 (NF2)-associated tumors.[4–6] Novel systemic medical treatments are needed to improve overall outcomes in patients with skull base tumors.

[a] Gilbert Family Neurofibromatosis Institute, Children's National Hospital, 111 Michigan Avenue Northwest, Washington, DC 20010, USA; [b] Department of Pediatric Hematology-Oncology; [c] Center for Genetics Research, Children's National Hospital, 111 Michigan Avenue Northwest, Washington, DC 20010, USA
* Corresponding author. Children's National Hospital, 111 Michigan Avenue Northwest, Washington, DC 20010.
E-mail address: mbornhorst@childrensnational.org

Otolaryngol Clin N Am 54 (2021) 789–801
https://doi.org/10.1016/j.otc.2021.05.004 oto.theclinics.com
0030-6665/21/

Over the past several decades, studies of the genome and tumor microenvironment have provided information regarding biological aberrations that are necessary for the growth and maintenance of tumors.[7–11] These studies have led to the development and initiation of clinical trials incorporating biological treatments of many skull base tumors (**Table 1**). This article focuses on advances in biological treatments of VSs in NF2 patients, meningiomas, chordomas, paragangliomas, and ELSTs.

TUMOR MOLECULAR PATHWAYS

Vestibular Schwannomas and Meningiomas

NF2, previously known as bilateral acoustic neurofibromatosis or central neurofibromatosis, is a multiple neoplasia syndrome that results from inactivating alterations in the *NF2* tumor suppressor gene on chromosome 22q12.[12,13] NF2 affects approximately 1 in 30,000 individuals worldwide and is inherited in an autosomal dominant pattern.[12,14] NF2 has a wide phenotypic variability, with nearly 100% penetrance by 60 years of age.[12,14] Patients present with a spectrum of nervous system tumors, including cranial and peripheral nerve schwannomas, meningiomas, and spinal ependymomas.[13]

VSs are benign tumors arising from Schwann cells of the eighth cranial nerve.[13] VSs are the most common tumor of the cerebellopontine angle and the fourth most common intracranial tumor in humans. They can be either isolated (95%; unilateral) or associated with NF2 (primarily bilateral).[15] They are the most common brain tumor affecting individuals with NF2, observed in 90% to 95% of patients, and serve as a primary diagnostic criteria for NF2.[12] Due to the anatomic location of VSs, patients present with hearing loss, tinnitus, imbalance, or a combination of these 3 symptoms.[16]

Meningiomas arise from the meningeal layer of the brain or spinal cord.[17] Approximately 50% of meningiomas are located in the skull base, and they are the second most common tumor in individuals with NF2.[18,19] Symptoms related

Table 1
Summary of targeted treatments utilized in skull base tumors

Drug Class	Molecular Target	Molecular Agent	Tumor Types	References
Antiangiogenesis	VEGF	Bevacizumab	VS, meningioma, chordoma	37–45,47
		Sunitinib	Meningioma, paraganglioma	10,49,50
	VEGF, PDGFR	Vatalanib	Meningioma	52
	VEGF, PDGFR, KIT	Pazopanib	ELST	51
	Fibroblast growth factor (likely)	IFN-α	Meningioma	82,83
TKIs	EGFR, ErbB2	Lapatinib	VS, chordoma	56,58
	MET, ALK, Ros-1	Crizotinib	VS	NCT04283669
	EGFR	Erlotinib, gefitinib, Cetuximab	VS, chordoma, meningioma	7,67–71
	PDGFR	Imatinib	Meningioma, chordoma	10,72
mTOR inhibitors	mTORC1	Everolimus (RAD001)	VS, paraganglioma, meningioma	74–78,80
	mTORC1/2	Sirolimus (rapamycin)	Chordoma	79

to meningiomas depend on their location and often are slow in onset. Clinical symptoms of headache due to increased intracranial pressure, focal neurologic (including cranial nerve) deficits, or generalized and partial seizures caused by focal mass effect are typical.[17]

NF2-associated tumors arise from inactivating mutations of the *NF2* gene encoding for the protein Merlin, also known as neurofibromin 2 or schwannomin.[20] Merlin interacts with other intracellular signaling pathways, including Hippo-YAP, cAMP/protein kinase A, FAK/Src, PI3K/AKT, Rac/PAK/JNK, WNT/B-catenin, integrins, receptor tyrosine kinase (RTK), Ras/MAPK, PAK, CD44, and Rac/Rho.[20,21] Through inactivation of these pathways, NF2-associated tumors have dysregulation of cell fate, proliferation, and survival. Disruption of the Hippo pathway results in YAP activation in human VSs, and loss of NF2/Merlin leads to increased nuclear YAP expression and cell proliferation in meningiomas and peripheral schwannomas, implying that the Hippo-YAP pathway also is a key component of meningioma and schwannoma development.[22,23] Key signaling molecules targeted in current biologically targeted therapeutic trials for VSs include Hippo-YAP, Ras/Rac, c-MET, epidermal growth factor receptor (EGFR), vascular endothelial growth factor (VEGF), CD44, mammalian target of rapamycin complex (mTORC) 1/2, and RTKs (**Table 2**). Interferon-alpha (IFN-α) and somatostatin receptor agonists, which target the tumor immune response and hormone receptors, also have been used for meningiomas (**Table 3**).[24]

Paragangliomas and Endolymphatic Sac Tumors

von Hippel–Lindau disease (VHL) is an autosomal dominant syndrome, which occurs secondary to germline mutations in the *VHL* tumor suppressor gene, located on chromosome 3.[25] VHL is seen in approximately 1 in 36,000 live births and is characterized by the presence of benign and malignant tumors, such as hemangioblastomas of the brain, spinal cord, and retina; pheochromocytoma and paraganglioma; renal cell carcinoma; neuroendocrine tumors; and ELSTs.[25] The primary skull base tumors associated with VHL are ELSTs and paragangliomas. ELSTs develop from endolymphatic epithelium within the vestibular aqueduct.[26] These tumors invade into the temporal bone and can cause hearing loss, tinnitus, vertigo, aural fullness, and facial-nerve dysfunction.[26,27] ELSTs are found in 6% to 15% of VHL patients and are rare in the general population.[27] These tumors have been treated primarily with agents that target the kinase signal pathway.[9]

Hereditary pheochromocytoma/paraganglioma syndrome (HPP) predisposes patients to the development of paragangliomas, pheochromocytomas, gastrointestinal stromal tumors, and pituitary adenomas.[28] Most patients with HPP harbor a mutation in a *SDHx* gene (*SDHA*, *SDHB*, *SDHC*, *SDHD*, and *SDHAF2*).[28,29] Paragangliomas are tumors of neural crest origin.[29] Patients with *SDHD*, *SDHC*, and *SCHAF2* variants are most likely to have skull base and neck paragangliomas, and screening guidelines for these patients may include dedicated imaging of the head and neck region along with whole-body magnetic resonance imaging (MRI) to improve resolution in this region.[28,29]

There are 2 primary signal pathways associated with paraganglioma development; hypoxia-associated signal pathway and kinase signal pathway.[30] Tumors with alterations in the *SDHx*, *VHL*, *FH*, *PDH2*, or *HIF2A* are associated primarily with alterations in the hypoxia-related pathway (cluster 1) whereas tumors with alterations in *RET* (can be associated with multiple endocrine neoplasia type 2), *MAX*, *TMEM127*, *KIF1Bβ*, and *NF1* (cluster 2) are associated with alterations in the kinase signaling pathway.[8]

Table 2
Clinical trials of biologic treatments of vestibular schwannomas

Investigators	Drugs Investigated	Partial Response	Stable Response	Progression	Audiological Outcomes
Alanin et al,[39] 2015; Plotkin et al,[37] 2012; Blakeley, et al,[40] 2016; Morris et al,[41] 2016; Farschtschi et al,[42] 2015; Goutagny and Kalamarides,[38] 2018; Hochart et al,[43] 2015; Sverak et al,[44] 2019	Bevacizumab	41% (95% CI, 31%–51%; *P*-effect < 0.01)[a]	47% (95% CI, 39%–55%; *P*-effect <0.01)[a]	7% (95% CI, 1%–15%; *P*-effect <0.01)[a]	Improvement: 20% (95% CI, 9%–33%; *P*-effect < 0.01) Stable: 69% (95% CI, 51%–85%; *P*-effect <0.01) Worse: 6% (95% CI, 1%–15%; *P*-effect = 0.01)
Plotkin et al,[45] 2019	Bevacizumab	37% (95% CI, 24%–52%) Overall response	71% of target and 50% nontarget VSs	0% target and 11% nontarget VSs	Hearing response in 39% (95% CI, 24%–56%) of evaluable ears. Decline in 9% of target (0 nontarget) ears
Karajannis et al,[74] 2014; Goutagny et al,[75] 2015; Goutagny et al,[76] 2017	RAD001	Karajannis et al—no objective responses	Goutagny et al—potential for stabilization		No objective responses
Karajannis et al,[56] 2012	Lapatinib	23.5%			30.8%

[a] Summary of 8 studies (Lu et al, 2019).[11]

Table 3
.Clinical trials of biologic treatments for meningiomas

Investigators	Drugs Investigated	Progression-free Survival
Karajannis et al,[77] 2014	mTORC	No response (monotherapy)
Grimm et al,[47] 2015; Kaley et al,[49] 2015; Raizer et al,[52] 2014	VEGF inhibitors	Grade I—up to 87% Grade II/III—37.5%–46% (grade II only up to 77%)
Norden et al,[69] 2010; Wen et al,[72] 2009	EGFR/PDGFR	EGFR—25% grade I, 29% grade II/III PDGFR—45% grade I, 0% grade II and higher
Chamberlain,[82] 2013; Chamberlain and Glantz,[83] 2008	IFN-α	Grade I—54% Grade II and higher—17%

Chordomas

Chordomas typically are located in the middle and posterior skull base compartments. They originate from extradural vestiges of the notochord and have a benign histopathology but exhibit aggressive clinical behavior with invasive and metastatic potential.[31] Studies show that many chordomas have dysregulation of the kinase signaling pathway, including platelet-derived growth factor receptor (PDGFR), EGFR, human ErbB2 (HER2), c-Met, and downstream PI3K/AKT and mammalian target of rapamyoin (mTOR).[32]

BIOLOGICAL THERAPY FOR SKULL BASE TUMORS

Biological therapy allows for a personalized approach to treatment by utilizing drugs designed to target unique genetic, epigenetic, or microenvironment alterations specific to cancer cells without affecting normal cells.[33] By targeting specific molecular pathways within the tumor, molecularly targeted therapies are being studied in patients with skull base tumors through clinical trials, with some showing promise in a subset of patients (see **Tables 2** and **3**). This section reviews promising molecularly targeted therapies for patients with NF2-associated (VSs and meningiomas) and other skull base tumors.

Bevacizumab/Vascular Endothelial Growth Factor Inhibitors

Bevacizumab is the first antiangiogenesis drug to receive Food and Drug Administration (FDA) approval.[34] It is a monoclonal antibody that inhibits VEGF, a main protein involved in inducing angiogenesis. Bevacizumab has been shown to slow or halt VS growth and even may improve hearing in some patients with NF2 (see **Table 2**).[11,35–44] A recently published multicenter phase 2 and biomarker study found that standard-dose bevacizumab (5 mg/kg every 3 weeks) was equally effective as high-dose bevacizumab (10 mg/kg every 2 weeks) for treatment of patients with NF2 VSs and hearing loss.[45] Although adults had notable tumor shrinkage following high-dose bevacizumab therapy, pediatric patients did not, suggesting that bevacizumab may not be an ideal first-line therapy for children with progressive VSs.[45]

Meningiomas and chordomas also up-regulate expression of VEGF.[8,9,46] When used in combination with surgery and RT, bevacizumab showed efficacy against a subset of recurrent meningiomas in a phase II clinical trial that had 6-month progression free survival (PFS-6) of 87%, 77%, and 46% in grades I, II, and III tumors, respectively (see **Table 3**).[47] Bevacizumab, in combination with erlotinib (inhibitor of EGFR), also has resulted in stability in a small study of 3 patients with chordomas (2 with skull base tumors).[48]

Sunitinib is a small molecule inhibitor of VEGF and multiple other pathways that had a PFS-6 of 42% in a phase II trial of 36 patients with grade II/III refractory meningioma (see **Table 3**).[49] Unfortunately, toxicity was common and up to 60% of patients had severe adverse events. The level of tumor expression of VEGF receptor 2 was predictive of response to sunitinib in this trial.[49] Preclinical and early clinical studies also suggest that sunitinib may be beneficial for patients with paragangliomas, although further studies are needed to determine which patients are most likely to benefit from this treatment.[10,50] Pazopanib, an inhibitor of VEGF, PDGF, and KIT, has been used successfully in a patient with ELST, which may lead to further trials in other patients with VHL-associated tumors.[9,51] Another trial using a VEGF small molecule inhibitor, vatalanib, resulted in a PFS-6 of 37.5% in a phase study of 22 patients with recurrent high-grade meningioma.[52]

Tyrosine Kinase Inhibitors

Lapatinib temporarily inhibits EGFR and ErbB2 by blocking phosphorylation and activation of Erk1/2 and Akt.[53] It was approved by the FDA in 2007 for use in the treatment of ErbB2 (HER2) overexpressing advanced or metastatic breast cancer in combination with chemotherapy.[53,54] Recent studies have suggested that abnormal activation of RTKs, such as those in the EGFR (or ErbB) family, may be of key importance in determining how Merlin controls cell proliferation.[55,56] EGFR and ErbB2 are overexpressed and activated in VSs, and lapatinib has antitumor activity in a preclinical schwannoma model.[57] These preclinical data led to the development of a phase 2 clinical trial evaluating lapatinib in patients with NF2 (NCT00973739).[56] Lapatinib generally was well tolerated, and volumetric (≥15% in volume reduction), and audiological response rates were 23.5% and 30.8%, respectively (see **Table 2**).[56] Lapatinib also has been used in clinical trials for chordomas, with a phase 2 trial in adults showing a clinical benefit rate (complete response + partial response + stable disease ≥6 months) of 22%.[58] Although encouraging, additional studies are required to fully understand the benefit of lapatinib for the management of these tumors.

Merlin interacts with CD44 and inhibits signaling through the MET proto-oncogene, an RTK.[59] VSs with an *NF2* mutation demonstrate dysregulation of MET expression and other associated genes.[59–61] Crizotinib (PF-2341066) is an FDA-approved drug that is a potent inhibitor of MET, ALK, and Ros-1.[62] Based on preclinical evidence, there is a current phase II clinical trial (NCT04283669) in the United States that is actively recruiting, using crizotinib for the treatment of progressive VSs.[61]

Several other tyrosine kinase inhibitors (TKIs) also are being studied for their effectiveness in the treatment of skull base tumors. Erlotinib is an oral EGFR TKI approved by the FDA for treatment of non–small cell lung cancer and pancreatic cancer.[63,64] Preclinical and clinical studies indicate that erlotinib crosses the blood-brain barrier in clinically active concentrations.[65,66] Erlotinib has been used in patients with NF2-associated VSs and chordomas showing some clinical benefit in patients with chordomas but minimal benefit in patients with VSs.[7,10,67,68] For meningiomas, single-arm phase II trials of the EGFR inhibitors, erlotinib and gefitinib, demonstrated PFS-6 of 25% for recurrent grade I and 29% for recurrent grade II/III tumors (see **Table 3**).[69] Case studies of cetuximab and gefitinib in patients with metastatic chondromas also showed response, with up to 44% tumor volume reduction in 1 study.[70,71] A phase II trial of the PDGFR inhibitor imatinib showed a PFS-6 of 45% for recurrent grade I meningioma, but unfortunately the PFS-6 was 0% for higher-grade tumors (see **Table 3**).[72] Imatinib trials for patients with chordomas have shown little benefit, with only a few patients showing partial response.[10] The TKI group as a whole are promising in the future treatment of NF2 associated tumors. Although some TKIs have shown promise as monotherapy, there is a movement to combine TKIs with each other or other forms of targeted therapy when treating skull base tumors.

Mammalian Target of Rapamycin Complex Inhibitors

Preclinical data in mice showed that mTORC1 inhibition delayed growth of NF2 schwannomas.[73] Based on this evidence, several recent clinical trials have been designed to study the effect of RAD001 (an mTORC1 inhibitor) in the treatment of VSs. None of the 9 patients with evaluable disease in 1 trial (NCT01419639) experienced a clinical or MRI response, and the study was closed according to predefined stopping rules[74] (see **Table 2**). Another study conducted in France (NCT01490476) duplicated these findings and did not reach their primary endpoint of 20% tumor volume reduction[75] (see **Table 2**). Secondary analysis looking at the rate of tumor growth pretreatment, post-treatment, and after the reintroduction of RAD001 suggested, however, the potential for RAD001 to stabilize or delay tumor growth.[75,76] Therefore, although mTOR inhibition has not proved to significantly decrease the size of NF2-associated VSs, there are potential benefits related to tumor stabilization and further studies may utilize mTOR inhibitors in combination with other targeted therapy.

The mTORC1/2 inhibitor everolimus did not show significant benefit in patients with NF2-associated meningiomas[77] (see **Table 3**). When used in combination with octreotide (a somatostatin analog), however, everolimus showed a PFS-6 of 55%, suggesting that this combination therapy may be active in patients with aggressive meningiomas (NCT02333565).[78] mTOR inhibitors (everolimus and rapamycin) also have been used for the treatment of paragangliomas (monotherapy) and chordomas (in combination with imatinib).[79,80] Similar to VSs, these studies did not show significant response.

Interferon-alpha

The mechanism action for interferons in tumors mostly is unknown, but this may be related to angiostatic properties.[81] Early studies determined that IFN-α shows some activity in patients with recurrent grade I but minimal activity in higher-grade (grade 2+) meningiomas, with studies demonstrating PFS-6 of 54% and 17%, respectively.[82,83] Studies to confirm these findings still need to be completed.

FUTURE DIRECTIONS

The current landscape of therapy for the treatment of skull base tumors and NF2 associated tumors includes the continued discovery of new agents specifically targeting the molecular pathways associated with specific tumors. The future of NF2 and other skull base clinical trials will need to focus on new agents that prevent drug resistance as well as combination therapy of agents targeting different components of the NF2 pathway. One example is the addition of MEK inhibitors to NF2-associated tumor treatment. MEK inhibitors target the Ras/Raf/MEK/ERK signaling pathway, inhibiting cell proliferation and inducing apoptosis.[84] There are compelling preclinical data suggesting that MEK inhibitors alone or in combination with other drugs (such as mTOR inhibitors) also could have a benefit in NF2 associated tumors.[85] Similarly, combination mTOR inhibitor plus TKI (ie, AZD2014 and the TKI dasatinib) was shown to prevent growth of VS cells in vitro and tumors in vivo for VSs.[86] In meningiomas, vismodegib (a smoothened [SMO] inhibitor) and GSK2256098 (an inhibitor of FAK) are being tested in patients who have tumors harboring mutations in the SMO gene and the NF2 gene (NCT02523014).[17]

SUMMARY

The treatment of skull base and NF2-associated tumors will require a multidisciplinary approach, using a combination of surgery, RT, and novel molecularly targeted therapies for optimal outcomes. Preclinical discoveries are being translated to clinical models at a rapid pace, with many ongoing trials assessing the efficacy of novel therapies (see **Table 1**). The exciting developments of molecularly targeted therapy for the treatment of skull base tumors hopefully will continue to provide noninvasive therapeutic options for patients. Future analysis and continued scientific discovery of the pathways driving tumor development and progression will aide in the creation of new targeted therapies for all skull base tumors. These treatments have the potential to greatly improve outcomes in patients NF2-associated and other skull base tumors.

CLINICS CARE POINTS

- Resent research studies have advanced understanding of the biological pathways required for growth and development of some skull base tumors.
- Molecularly targeted therapies for patients with NF2-associated and other skull base tumors show promise in recent clinical trials.
- Additional clinical trials can help identify promising new systemic therapies that can be used either alone or in combination with surgery and RT in patients with skull base tumors.

DISCLOSURE

There are no relevant commercial or financial interests to disclose. M. Bornhorst has served as a consultant for AstraZeneca, but this is not felt to be a conflict of interest related to the information presented in this article. There are no funding sources relevant to this article.

REFERENCES

1. Hudgins PA, Baugnon KL. Head and Neck: Skull Base Imaging. Neurosurgery 2018;82(3):255–67.
2. Mazzoni A, Krengli M. Historical development of the treatment of skull base tumours. Rep Pract Oncol Radiother 2016;21(4):319–24.
3. DeMonte F. Management considerations for malignant tumors of the skull base. J Neurooncol 2020;150(3):361–5.
4. Wagenmann M, Scheckenbach K, Kraus B, et al. [Complications of anterior skull base surgery]. HNO 2018;66(6):438–46.
5. Couldwell WT, Fukushima T, Giannotta SL, et al. Petroclival meningiomas: surgical experience in 109 cases. J Neurosurg 1996;84(1):20–8.
6. Seferis C, Torrens M, Paraskevopoulou C, et al. Malignant transformation in vestibular schwannoma: report of a single case, literature search, and debate. J Neurosurg 2014;121(Suppl):160–6.
7. Di Maio S, Yip S, Al Zhrani GA, et al. Novel targeted therapies in chordoma: an update. Ther Clin Risk Manag 2015;11:873–83.
8. Liu Y, Liu L, Zhu F. Therapies targeting the signal pathways of pheochromocytoma and paraganglioma. Onco Targets Ther 2019;12:7227–41.

9. Nelson T, Hu J, Bannykh S, et al. Clinical response to pazopanib in a patient with endolymphatic sac tumor not associated with von Hippel-Lindau syndrome. CNS Oncol 2020;9(1):CNS50.
10. Meng T, Jin J, Jiang C, et al. Molecular Targeted Therapy in the Treatment of Chordoma: A Systematic Review. Front Oncol 2019;9:30.
11. Lu VM, Ravindran K, Graffeo CS, et al. Efficacy and safety of bevacizumab for vestibular schwannoma in neurofibromatosis type 2: a systematic review and meta-analysis of treatment outcomes. J Neurooncol 2019;144(2):239–48.
12. Asthagiri AR, Parry DM, Butman JA, et al. Neurofibromatosis type 2. Lancet 2009; 373(9679):1974–86.
13. Coy S, Rashid R, Stemmer-Rachamimov A, et al. An update on the CNS manifestations of neurofibromatosis type 2. Acta Neuropathol 2020;139(4):643–65.
14. Evans DG, Moran A, King A, et al. Incidence of vestibular schwannoma and neurofibromatosis 2 in the North West of England over a 10-year period: higher incidence than previously thought. Otol Neurotol 2005;26(1):93–7.
15. Yao L, Alahmari M, Temel Y, et al. Therapy of Sporadic and NF2-related vestibular schwannoma. Cancers (Basel) 2020;12(4):835.
16. Campian J, Gutmann DH. CNS tumors in neurofibromatosis. J Clin Oncol 2017; 35(21):2378–85.
17. Buerki RA, Horbinski CM, Kruser T, et al. An overview of meningiomas. Future Oncol 2018;14(21):2161–77.
18. Kerr K, Qualmann K, Esquenazi Y, et al. Familial syndromes involving meningiomas provide mechanistic insight into sporadic disease. Neurosurgery 2018; 83(6):1107–18.
19. Nanda A, Vannemreddy P. Recurrence and outcome in skull base meningiomas: do they differ from other intracranial meningiomas? Skull Base 2008;18(4): 243–52.
20. Okada T, You L, Giancotti FG. Shedding light on Merlin's wizardry. Trends Cell Biol 2007;17(5):222–9.
21. Hamaratoglu F, Willecke M, Kango-Singh M, et al. The tumour-suppressor genes NF2/Merlin and Expanded act through Hippo signalling to regulate cell proliferation and apoptosis. Nat Cell Biol 2006;8(1):27–36.
22. Striedinger K, VandenBerg SR, Baia GS, et al. The neurofibromatosis 2 tumor suppressor gene product, merlin, regulates human meningioma cell growth by signaling through YAP. Neoplasia 2008;10(11):1204–12.
23. Zhao F, Yang Z, Chen Y, et al. Deregulation of the hippo pathway promotes tumor cell proliferation through yap activity in human sporadic vestibular schwannoma. World Neurosurg 2018;117:e269–79.
24. Karsy M, Guan J, Cohen A, et al. Medical management of meningiomas: current status, failed treatments, and promising horizons. Neurosurg Clin N Am 2016; 27(2):249–60.
25. Findeis-Hosey JJ, McMahon KQ, Findeis SK. Von Hippel-Lindau disease. J Pediatr Genet 2016;5(2):116–23.
26. Shanbhogue KP, Hoch M, Fatterpaker G, et al. von Hippel-Lindau disease: review of genetics and imaging. Radiol Clin North Am 2016;54(3):409–22.
27. Kim HJ, Butman JA, Brewer C, et al. Tumors of the endolymphatic sac in patients with von Hippel-Lindau disease: implications for their natural history, diagnosis, and treatment. J Neurosurg 2005;102(3):503–12.
28. Rednam SP, Erez A, Druker H, et al. Von Hippel-Lindau and hereditary pheochromocytoma/paraganglioma syndromes: clinical features, genetics, and surveillance recommendations in childhood. Clin Cancer Res 2017;23(12):e68–75.

29. Muth A, Crona J, Gimm O, et al. Genetic testing and surveillance guidelines in hereditary pheochromocytoma and paraganglioma. J Intern Med 2019;285(2):187–204.
30. Pillai S, Gopalan V, Smith RA, et al. Updates on the genetics and the clinical impacts on phaeochromocytoma and paraganglioma in the new era. Crit Rev Oncol Hematol 2016;100:190–208.
31. George B, Bresson D, Herman P, et al. Chordomas: a review. Neurosurg Clin N Am 2015;26(3):437–52.
32. Tamborini E, Virdis E, Negri T, et al. Analysis of receptor tyrosine kinases (RTKs) and downstream pathways in chordomas. Neuro Oncol 2010;12(8):776–89.
33. Chae YK, Pan AP, Davis AA, et al. Path toward precision oncology: review of targeted therapy studies and tools to aid in defining "actionability" of a molecular lesion and patient management support. Mol Cancer Ther 2017;16(12):2645–55.
34. Goodman L. Persistence–luck–Avastin. J Clin Invest 2004;113(7):934.
35. Killeen DE, Klesse L, Tolisano AM, et al. Long-term effects of bevacizumab on vestibular schwannoma volume in neurofibromatosis type 2 patients. J Neurol Surg B Skull Base 2019;80(5):540–6.
36. Plotkin SR, Stemmer-Rachamimov AO, Barker FG 2nd, et al. Hearing improvement after bevacizumab in patients with neurofibromatosis type 2. N Engl J Med 2009;361(4):358–67.
37. Plotkin SR, Merker VL, Halpin C, et al. Bevacizumab for progressive vestibular schwannoma in neurofibromatosis type 2: a retrospective review of 31 patients. Otol Neurotol 2012;33(6):1046–52.
38. Goutagny S, Kalamarides M. Medical treatment in neurofibromatosis type 2. Review of the literature and presentation of clinical reports. Neurochirurgie 2018;64(5):370–4.
39. Alanin MC, Klausen C, Caye-Thomasen P, et al. The effect of bevacizumab on vestibular schwannoma tumour size and hearing in patients with neurofibromatosis type 2. Eur Arch Otorhinolaryngol 2015;272(12):3627–33.
40. Blakeley JO, Ye X, Duda DG, et al. Efficacy and Biomarker Study of Bevacizumab for Hearing Loss Resulting From Neurofibromatosis Type 2-Associated Vestibular Schwannomas. J Clin Oncol 2016;34(14):1669–75.
41. Morris KA, Golding JF, Axon PR, et al. Bevacizumab in neurofibromatosis type 2 (NF2) related vestibular schwannomas: a nationally coordinated approach to delivery and prospective evaluation. Neurooncol Pract 2016;3(4):281–9.
42. Farschtschi S, Kollmann P, Dalchow C, et al. Reduced dosage of bevacizumab in treatment of vestibular schwannomas in patients with neurofibromatosis type 2. Eur Arch Otorhinolaryngol 2015;272(12):3857–60.
43. Hochart A, Gaillard V, Baroncini M, et al. Bevacizumab decreases vestibular schwannomas growth rate in children and teenagers with neurofibromatosis type 2. J Neurooncol 2015;124(2):229–36.
44. Sverak P, Adams ME, Haines SJ, et al. Bevacizumab for hearing preservation in neurofibromatosis type 2: emphasis on patient-reported outcomes and toxicities. Otolaryngol Head Neck Surg 2019;160(3):526–32.
45. Plotkin SR, Duda DG, Muzikansky A, et al. Multicenter, prospective, phase II and biomarker study of high-dose bevacizumab as induction therapy in patients with neurofibromatosis type 2 and progressive vestibular schwannoma. J Clin Oncol 2019;37(35):3446–54.
46. Le Rhun E, Taillibert S, Chamberlain MC. Systemic therapy for recurrent meningioma. Expert Rev Neurother 2016;16(8):889–901.

47. Grimm S, Kumthekar P, Chamberlain M, et al. MNGO-04: phase II trial of bevacizumab in patients with surgery and radiation refractory progressive meningioma. Neuro Oncol 2015;17(Suppl 5):v130.
48. Asklund T, Sandstrom M, Shahidi S, et al. Durable stabilization of three chordoma cases by bevacizumab and erlotinib. Acta Oncol 2014;53(7):980–4.
49. Kaley TJ, Wen P, Schiff D, et al. Phase II trial of sunitinib for recurrent and progressive atypical and anaplastic meningioma. Neuro Oncol 2015;17(1):116–21.
50. Ayala-Ramirez M, Chougnet CN, Habra MA, et al. Treatment with sunitinib for patients with progressive metastatic pheochromocytomas and sympathetic paragangliomas. J Clin Endocrinol Metab 2012;97(11):4040–50.
51. Harris PA, Boloor A, Cheung M, et al. Discovery of 5-[[4-[(2,3-dimethyl-2H-indazol-6-yl)methylamino]-2-pyrimidinyl]amino]-2-methyl-b enzenesulfonamide (Pazopanib), a novel and potent vascular endothelial growth factor receptor inhibitor. J Med Chem 2008;51(15):4632–40.
52. Raizer JJ, Grimm SA, Rademaker A, et al. A phase II trial of PTK787/ZK 222584 in recurrent or progressive radiation and surgery refractory meningiomas. J Neurooncol 2014;117(1):93–101.
53. Medina PJ, Goodin S. Lapatinib: a dual inhibitor of human epidermal growth factor receptor tyrosine kinases. Clin Ther 2008;30(8):1426–47.
54. Mukherjee A, Dhadda AS, Shehata M, et al. Lapatinib: a tyrosine kinase inhibitor with a clinical role in breast cancer. Expert Opin Pharmacother 2007;8(13):2189–204.
55. Ahmad ZK, Brown CM, Cueva RA, et al. ErbB expression, activation, and inhibition with lapatinib and tyrphostin (AG825) in human vestibular schwannomas. Otol Neurotol 2011;32(5):841–7.
56. Karajannis MA, Legault G, Hagiwara M, et al. Phase II trial of lapatinib in adult and pediatric patients with neurofibromatosis type 2 and progressive vestibular schwannomas. Neuro Oncol 2012;14(9):1163–70.
57. Ammoun S, Cunliffe CH, Allen JC, et al. ErbB/HER receptor activation and preclinical efficacy of lapatinib in vestibular schwannoma. Neuro Oncol 2010; 12(8):834–43.
58. Stacchiotti S, Tamborini E, Lo Vullo S, et al. Phase II study on lapatinib in advanced EGFR-positive chordoma. Ann Oncol 2013;24(7):1931–6.
59. Morrison H, Sherman LS, Legg J, et al. The NF2 tumor suppressor gene product, merlin, mediates contact inhibition of growth through interactions with CD44. Genes Dev 2001;15(8):968–80.
60. Torres-Martin M, Lassaletta L, San-Roman-Montero J, et al. Microarray analysis of gene expression in vestibular schwannomas reveals SPP1/MET signaling pathway and androgen receptor deregulation. Int J Oncol 2013;42(3):848–62.
61. Troutman S, Moleirinho S, Kota S, et al. Crizotinib inhibits NF2-associated schwannoma through inhibition of focal adhesion kinase 1. Oncotarget 2016; 7(34):54515–25.
62. Cui JJ, Tran-Dube M, Shen H, et al. Structure based drug design of crizotinib (PF-02341066), a potent and selective dual inhibitor of mesenchymal-epithelial transition factor (c-MET) kinase and anaplastic lymphoma kinase (ALK). J Med Chem 2011;54(18):6342–63.
63. Johnson JR, Cohen M, Sridhara R, et al. Approval summary for erlotinib for treatment of patients with locally advanced or metastatic non-small cell lung cancer after failure of at least one prior chemotherapy regimen. Clin Cancer Res 2005; 11(18):6414–21.

64. Moore MJ, Goldstein D, Hamm J, et al. Erlotinib plus gemcitabine compared with gemcitabine alone in patients with advanced pancreatic cancer: a phase III trial of the National Cancer Institute of Canada Clinical Trials Group. J Clin Oncol 2007;25(15):1960–6.
65. Katayama T, Shimizu J, Suda K, et al. Efficacy of erlotinib for brain and leptomeningeal metastases in patients with lung adenocarcinoma who showed initial good response to gefitinib. J Thorac Oncol 2009;4(11):1415–9.
66. Meany HJ, Fox E, McCully C, et al. The plasma and cerebrospinal fluid pharmacokinetics of erlotinib and its active metabolite (OSI-420) after intravenous administration of erlotinib in non-human primates. Cancer Chemother Pharmacol 2008; 62(3):387–92.
67. Plotkin SR, Halpin C, McKenna MJ, et al. Erlotinib for progressive vestibular schwannoma in neurofibromatosis 2 patients. Otol Neurotol 2010;31(7):1135–43.
68. Lebellec L, Chauffert B, Blay JY, et al. Advanced chordoma treated by first-line molecular targeted therapies: Outcomes and prognostic factors. A retrospective study of the French Sarcoma Group (GSF/GETO) and the Association des Neuro-Oncologues d'Expression Francaise (ANOCEF). Eur J Cancer 2017;79:119–28.
69. Norden AD, Raizer JJ, Abrey LE, et al. Phase II trials of erlotinib or gefitinib in patients with recurrent meningioma. J Neurooncol 2010;96(2):211–7.
70. Hof H, Welzel T, Debus J. Effectiveness of cetuximab/gefitinib in the therapy of a sacral chordoma. Onkologie 2006;29(12):572–4.
71. Linden O, Stenberg L, Kjellen E. Regression of cervical spinal cord compression in a patient with chordoma following treatment with cetuximab and gefitinib. Acta Oncol 2009;48(1):158–9.
72. Wen PY, Yung WK, Lamborn KR, et al. Phase II study of imatinib mesylate for recurrent meningiomas (North American Brain Tumor Consortium study 01-08). Neuro Oncol 2009;11(6):853–60.
73. Giovannini M, Bonne NX, Vitte J, et al. mTORC1 inhibition delays growth of neurofibromatosis type 2 schwannoma. Neuro Oncol 2014;16(4):493–504.
74. Karajannis MA, Legault G, Hagiwara M, et al. Phase II study of everolimus in children and adults with neurofibromatosis type 2 and progressive vestibular schwannomas. Neuro Oncol 2014;16(2):292–7.
75. Goutagny S, Raymond E, Esposito-Farese M, et al. Phase II study of mTORC1 inhibition by everolimus in neurofibromatosis type 2 patients with growing vestibular schwannomas. J Neurooncol 2015;122(2):313–20.
76. Goutagny S, Giovannini M, Kalamarides M. A 4-year phase II study of everolimus in NF2 patients with growing vestibular schwannomas. J Neurooncol 2017; 133(2):443–5.
77. Karajannis M, Osorio D, Filatov A, et al. AT-30: effects of everolimus on meningioma growth in patients with neurofibromatosis type 2. Neuro Oncol 2014; 16(Suppl 5):v15.
78. Graillon T, Sanson M, Campello C, et al. Everolimus and octreotide for patients with recurrent meningioma: results from the phase II CEVOREM trial. Clin Cancer Res 2020;26(3):552–7.
79. Stacchiotti S, Marrari A, Tamborini E, et al. Response to imatinib plus sirolimus in advanced chordoma. Ann Oncol 2009;20(11):1886–94.
80. Oh DY, Kim TW, Park YS, et al. Phase 2 study of everolimus monotherapy in patients with nonfunctioning neuroendocrine tumors or pheochromocytomas/paragangliomas. Cancer 2012;118(24):6162–70.
81. Dorr RT. Interferon-alpha in malignant and viral diseases. A Review. Drugs 1993; 45(2):177–211.

82. Chamberlain MC. IFN-alpha for recurrent surgery- and radiation-refractory high-grade meningioma: a retrospective case series. CNS Oncol 2013;2(3):227–35.
83. Chamberlain MC, Glantz MJ. Interferon-alpha for recurrent World Health Organization grade 1 intracranial meningiomas. Cancer 2008;113(8):2146–51.
84. Cheng Y, Tian H. Current development status of MEK inhibitors. Molecules 2017; 22(10):1551.
85. Fuse MA, Dinh CT, Vitte J, et al. Preclinical assessment of MEK1/2 inhibitors for neurofibromatosis type 2-associated schwannomas reveals differences in efficacy and drug resistance development. Neuro Oncol 2019;21(4):486–97.
86. Sagers JE, Beauchamp RL, Zhang Y, et al. Combination therapy with mTOR kinase inhibitor and dasatinib as a novel therapeutic strategy for vestibular schwannoma. Sci Rep 2020;10(1):4211.

Biologics for Immune-Mediated Sensorineural Hearing Loss

Andrea Vambutas, MD*, Daniella V. Davia

KEYWORDS

- Autoimmmune inner ear disease (AIED) • Interleukin-1 (IL-1)
- Tumor necrosis factor (TNF) • Corticosteroids

KEY POINTS

- Corticosteroids should be the initial treatment for immune-mediated hearing losses.
- Corticosteroids modulate tumor necrosis factor levels.
- Inhibition of interleukin-1 may be beneficial in corticosteroid-resistant autoimmune inner ear disease.

BACKGROUND AND DEFINITIONS

Immune-mediated hearing loss (IMED) encompasses several disease processes. The definition of immune-mediated hearing loss would be any sensorineural hearing loss that responds to an immunomodulatory drug (**Table 1**). Therefore, sudden sensorineural hearing loss (SSNHL), autoimmune inner ear disease (AIED) and Meniere's disease could be classified as immune-mediated hearing losses. Historically, corticosteroid responsiveness defined immune-mediated hearing loss.[1] However, we recently identified that corticosteroid-resistant patients with AIED responded favorably to interleukin-1 (IL-1) inhibition, thereby suggesting that the definition of immune-mediated hearing loss be extended to patients who respond to immunomodulators, not exclusively corticosteroids.[2] Indeed, the natural history of AIED is that although 70% of patients respond to corticosteroids initially, after 3 years, responsiveness declines to 14%.[3] Frequently these diseases can be clearly defined, as in the case of SSNHL, where an acute decline in hearing is rapid, unilateral, and isolated. However, when the disease process recurs, many practitioners use terms of AIED and cochlear Meniere's disease interchangeably, and describe the acute event as an SSNHL. Given that 50% of episodes of hearing decline in AIED may have concomitant vertigo,[4] it is possible that AIED and Meniere's disease may represent a

Department of Otolaryngology, Zucker School of Medicine at Hofstra-Northwell, Hearing and Speech Center, 430 Lakeville Road, New Hyde Park, NY 11040, USA
* Corresponding author.
E-mail address: AVambuta@northwell.edu

Otolaryngol Clin N Am 54 (2021) 803–813
https://doi.org/10.1016/j.otc.2021.05.005
oto.theclinics.com

Table 1
Biologics used in immune-mediated hearing loss

Target	Drug Names
Tumor necrosis factor-α	Etanercept Infliximab Golimumab Corticosteroids N-acetylcysteine
Interleukin-1β	Anakinra Canakinumab Rilonacept
c-Jun N-terminal kinase	AM-111
Multiple targets	Mycophenolate mofetil Methotrexate Rituximab Cyclophosphamide

In memory of Vida K. Vambutas, PhD, a biochemist whose interest and insights into biologic mechanisms of disease elucidated new targets for therapeutic intervention.

continuum, especially in the instance of bilateral disease. In fact, several investigators have postulated that one etiology of Meniere's disease is autoimmune.[5,6]

PATHOGENESIS OF DISEASE

Inner ear inflammation is triggered by the release of cytokines from macrophages in response to unknown stimuli. These cytokines, in turn, dictate adaptive T-cell responses, and further result in T-cell polarization, further cytokine production, antibody formation, and cellular destruction, which is a basic mechanism in classic autoimmune diseases (**Fig. 1**). It is postulated that viral antigens, and self-antigens, may trigger immune responses. However, unlike many other autoimmune diseases, there is a paucity of robust autoantigens in AIED. Although correlations to HSP70, cochlin, P0, and other self-antigens have been described, these autoantigens are neither expressed in most of those with disease, nor is there clear evidence that they are pathogenic.

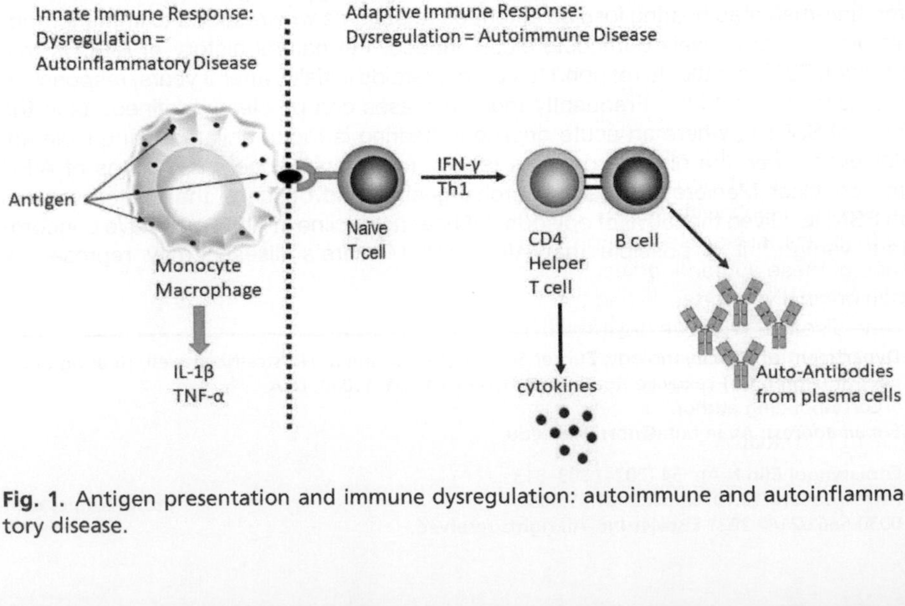

Fig. 1. Antigen presentation and immune dysregulation: autoimmune and autoinflammatory disease.

It is important to recognize a new class of immune-mediated disorders called autoinflammatory diseases, which is characterized by dysregulation of the innate immune system. Here, cytokine release is triggered by a single insult, rather than the classic 2 insults requisite for inflammatory cytokine release.[7] Autoinflammatory diseases are diseases of the innate immune system, and therefore, because they are mediated by monocytes, do not result in antibody production or T-cell responses.[8] The classic autoinflammatory disease is Muckle Wells disease,[9] which is the result of a gain-of-function mutation in the NLRP3 inflammasome and results in excessive IL-1β production by monocytes.[10] Muckle Wells clinically is characterized by sensorineural hearing loss, skin rashes, and uveitis.[9] Interestingly, the clinical features of Muckle Wells disease are similar to Cogan disease, which is classically corticosteroid responsive,[11] unlike Muckle Wells disease, which demonstrates poor response to corticosteroid therapy. Therefore, the role of IL-1β in the pathogenesis of sensorineural hearing loss becomes obvious through this monogenic disease process.[12]

CYTOKINES RELEASED BY THE INNATE IMMUNE SYSTEM AND BIOLOGIC TARGETING

Initiating events for inflammation is activation of the innate immune system in which monocytes, macrophages, and microglia release IL-1, tumor necrosis factor alpha (TNF-α), and other cytokines, thereby activating T cells and the innate immune system. The 2 major pathways that trigger inflammation in the inner ear are the TNF and IL-1 pathways that signal to c-Jun N-terminal kinase (JNK) In **Fig. 2**, the 2 pathways are shown, together with biologic agents that have been used clinically to block these cytokines and inflammatory mediators.

Fig. 2. Convergent pathways of inflammation and targets for inhibition.

Cell surface receptors for IL-1 type 1 receptor (IL-1R1) or TNF receptor binds their respective cytokines and initiates intracellular signaling. Disruption of either TNF or IL-1 from engagement of their cognate receptor has been used therapeutically to ameliorate various forms of immune-mediated hearing loss. Both pathways can converge to JNK, which has also served as a biologic target for therapeutic intervention for immune-mediated hearing loss. IL-1 type 2 receptor (IL-1R2) is a decoy receptor for IL-1 and can sequester IL-1 without initiating signaling. Decoy receptors for TNF exist; however, their role in immune-mediated hearing loss is unknown.

Classic autoimmune diseases result in T-cell polarization, and autoantibody production. Interestingly, to date, there is a lack of compelling evidence of autoantibody production in AIED. During the 1990s, the 68-kD antibody to heat shock protein emerged as a biomarker of steroid-sensitive immune-mediated hearing loss.[13] However, since that time, transfer of the 68-kD protein to animal models did not result in disease manifestation.[14] The other antibody identified was the anti-cochlin antibody in sera of patients with AIED.[15,16] Here, high-titer antibodies were identified, and transfer to an animal model recapitulated disease. Our laboratory further validated the presence of these autoantibodies; however, we observed these antibodies at a lower titer than originally reported,[17] and therefore potentially inconsistent with a classic autoimmune disease. What we did identify was a cross-reactivity between cochlin and some environmental molds, potentially identifying a mechanism for trigger of hearing decline in some patients based on exposure.[18]

CORTICOSTEROIDS

Corticosteroids have remained the first-line agent for any acute decline in hearing for SSNHL, since early studies that suggested hearing recovery was significantly better

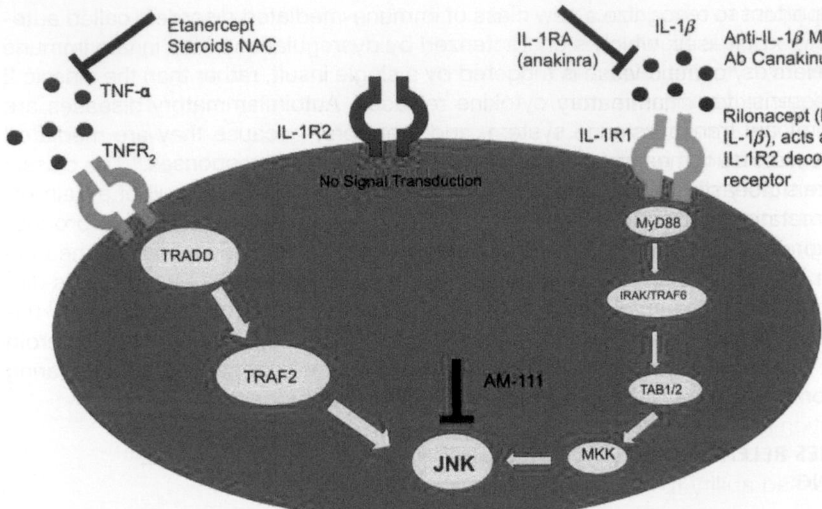

Fig. 2. Convergent pathways of inflammation and targets for inhibition.

with corticosteroids as compared with no treatment.[19,20] Historically, early studies suggested there is a high degree of spontaneous recovery of hearing within the first 14 days following the hearing loss.[21] Despite this, most practitioners advocate timely treatment is a requisite step toward hearing recovery, and substantial delays may result in a failure to respond. Interestingly, there has not been a compelling study that has clearly identified a timeline after which corticosteroid responsiveness is lost. Choice of corticosteroids have largely been for those that have larger glucocorticoid effects over mineralocorticoid effects, as the immunosuppressive activity is a result of the glucocorticoid effect.

DIFFERENCES IN STEROID-RESPONSIVE RATES BETWEEN VARIOUS FORMS OF IMMUNE-MEDIATED HEARING LOSS

Perhaps the most well-defined corticosteroid response rate is for SSNHL, in which the overall response rate is accepted to be approximately 60%.[19] Evaluation of treatment efficacy is complicated by the recognition that in those with mild-moderate SSNHL, there are cases of spontaneous recovery, unlike those with severe loss, in whom spontaneous recovery is significantly less likely. In this severe group, corticosteroid intervention was clearly superior to spontaneous recovery rates.[22] Moreover, in SSNHL, the method of delivery, oral or intratympanic, is comparable, as shown in the large multicentered clinical trial.[23] Combined use if oral and intratympanic may be superior, as demonstrated in a small study,[24] and was subsequently validated in a larger cohort.[25]

SSNHL and AIED have similar corticosteroid response rates at initial disease presentation of 60% to 70%. For patients with recurrent declines in hearing, such as AIED, although 60% to 70% of patients respond initially, the response rate declines over time.[3,26] This decline may be the result of T-cell polarization and enhanced cytokine production, which correlates with a poorer clinical prognosis.[27] Despite the noted decline over time, there is a subset of patients with AIED who are steroid dependent, in whom, upon weaning, the hearing declines further, necessitating increasing corticosteroid dose to maintain hearing. In these instances, switching to a steroid-sparing immunosuppressive has proven beneficial, as discussed later in this article. Furthermore, although it is highly unusual to identify patients with AIED with afflicted first-degree relatives, genetic variation in the gene POU4F3 has been described to result in steroid-sensitive immune-mediated hearing loss that is conferred through autosomal dominant transmission.[28] In addition, the reality is that most patients with fluctuating sensorineural hearing loss do not have afflicted first-degree relatives.

Meniere's disease has a significantly lower corticosteroid response rate of less than 50% for hearing improvement.[29] Corticosteroids have been shown to result in a significantly higher rate of vertigo control in Meniere's disease.[30] It is unclear as to why corticosteroids differentially affect vertigo and hearing recovery differently.

Quantification of the amount of hearing to be recovered in response to corticosteroids is surprisingly little in AIED. In the largest study to date, less than 10 dB pure tone average and less than 12% word recognition score was achieved after a 1 month trial of corticosteroids.[26] The mechanism by which corticosteroids work to reduce inflammation is likely multifactorial. We have previously shown in a large series of patients with immune-mediated hearing loss, elevated levels of TNF in plasma correlated with increased ability to respond favorably to corticosteroids.[31]

COMPLICATIONS OF CORTICOSTEROIDS

Corticosteroids are used frequently; however, despite frequent use, a myriad of complications are associated with their use. If administered orally, hypothalamic-pituitary-adrenal axis suppression, hypertension, hyperglycemia, bone fragility, and cataracts are the most worrisome complications.[32] Symptoms of adrenal crisis include hypotension, lethargy, hypoglycemia, hyponatremia, seizure and coma. Less worrisome, however, still of significant concern, include skin fragility, truncal obesity/cushingoid appearance, gastrointestinal disturbances, and mood instability. Although corticosteroids administered through the intratympanic route spares many of these systemic complications, local infection and/or tympanic membrane perforation may occur. Furthermore, a portion of the intratympanic steroids may still be absorbed systemically, and therefore blood glucose monitoring in the 24 hours postprocedure should still be undertaken.

TUMOR NECROSIS FACTOR ANTAGONISM

TNF antagonists have been tried to ameliorate immune-mediated hearing loss with variable, but limited success when administered systemically.[33,34] The rationale for use of TNF antagonists largely arose from the early studies in guinea pigs that demonstrated release of TNF in response to Keyhole limpet hemocyanin (KLH) challenge.[35] Despite these elegant studies, in patients given an initial trial of corticosteroids, the TNF antagonist etanercept was no better than placebo in maintaining hearing.[34] Similarly, response to systemic etanercept demonstrated a bell curve in an open-label study, with 30% responding, 57% no change, and 13% worsening.[33] Notably, in steroid-dependent patients, 2 small studies using 2 different TNF antagonists (infliximab and golimumab), administered via an intratympanic approach, were successful in weaning the patients off corticosteroids.[36,37] Cogan syndrome has been predominantly treated with corticosteroids,[38] although more recently, TNF antagonist therapy has been demonstrated to be beneficial in Cogan syndrome.[39]

ANTI-INTERLEUKIN-1 THERAPY

In patients with Muckle Wells syndrome and other autoinflammatory diseases, IL-1 inhibition results in significant amelioration of most symptoms, including skin rashes and ocular manifestations. Despite case reports of hearing improvement in response to IL-1 blockade,[40] most patents do not experience significant hearing improvement, although hearing stabilized with IL-1 blockade.[41] We initially discovered in patients with end-stage AIED undergoing cochlear implantation, that they differentially expressed the IL-1 decoy receptor (IL-1R2) in their peripheral blood immune cells in response to their autologous perilymph.[42] Based on these studies, we further identified that the decoy receptor was induced in corticosteroid-responsive patients with AIED; however, in corticosteroid-resistant patients, decoy receptor expression was elevated and could not be further induced. This correlated with elevated plasma levels of IL-1 in corticosteroid-resistant patients.[43] Our observations led to a small clinical trial for corticosteroid-resistant AIED, using the IL-1 inhibitor anakinra. Notably, hearing improvement was significant for both improvement in pure tone average and speech discrimination scores, and correlated with a reduction in plasma IL-1β.[2] These patients were subsequently sequenced and all found to be negative for the NLRP3 mutation that is associated with Muckle Wells syndrome.

METHOTREXATE

Methotrexate is an immunomodulator that has been used in AIED with limited success. Methotrexate is an antimetabolite drug that has been used extensively in multiple autoimmune diseases. Its mode of action is multiple, including inhibition of TNF, IL-1, increasing the regulatory cytokine IL-10, and inhibiting cytokines produced by T-cell activation, and altering the receptor activator of nuclear factor-kB ligand pathway.[44] It is unclear as to its mode of action in AIED, and actual effect on various proinflammatory cytokines. Methotrexate was identified to be no better than placebo in maintaining hearing post corticosteroids.[45] Methotrexate is largely used in combination with other agents in autoimmune diseases, and is rarely used as monotherapy, as efficacy is superior when combination therapy is used.[46]

C-JUN-N-TERMINAL KINASE ANTAGONISTS

Recently it became apparent that the downstream ligand, JNK ligands, demonstrated promise in the amelioration of SSNHL. JNK is the principal mechanism of cell death following cochlear inflammation.[47,48] In a phase II study, the JNK ligand, AM-111 was demonstrated to have a statistically significant effect on speech discrimination and tinnitus remission.[49] The phase III study did not achieve its primary endpoint; however, the post hoc analysis did demonstrate a treatment response in those patients with a profound SSNHL.[50]

MYCOPHENOLATE MOFETIL

Mycophenolate mofetil (MMF) is an immunosuppressive agent used in organ transplantation. It has been demonstrated to exert broad cytokine suppression in monocytes, including IL-1α, IL-1β, interferon-γ, and TNF.[51] It also decreases nitric oxide by inducible nitric oxide synthase.[52] Isolated case reports exist attesting to the use in Cogan syndrome and AIED. Given the paucity of controlled studies, it is unclear as to whether significant benefit can be derived in immune-mediated hearing loss.[53] Moreover, MMF is a teratogen and has been linked to microtia in 12 patients and external auditory canal atresia in 9.[54]

ANTIOXIDANTS

Antioxidants have been suggested to be beneficial in immune-mediated hearing losses and acoustic trauma. The most widely studied has been N-acetylcysteine (NAC).

NAC has been shown to improve corticosteroid outcomes when used in conjunction with oral corticosteroids in SSNHL.[55] We have identified that corticosteroid-responsive immune-mediated hearing loss is characterized by high TNF levels relative to those patients who do not respond.[31] Moreover, we have characterized that NAC inhibits TNF in vitro in these patients.[56] Interestingly, a clinical trial using NAC alone suggested it was superior to corticosteroids for hearing restoration.[57]

OTHER IMMUNOSUPPRESSIVE AGENTS

Classically, use of cyclophosphamide has been described in combination with corticosteroids for the treatment of AIED.[1] This agent has largely been abandoned because of systemic toxicity. Rituximab, an agent that depletes B cells, and therefore prevents autoantibody production, demonstrated a modest hearing benefit in a very small AIED cohort; however, further study is warranted to determine whether the response is durable.[58] There have been many case reports citing various immunosuppressive agents as beneficial in recovery of sensorineural hearing loss in isolation or in conjunction with a rare disease. Specifically, literature on Cogan syndrome, Susac syndrome, Muckle Wells syndrome, and POU4F3 mutations all have reports of use of various immunosuppressive agents correlating with hearing improvement. Similar reports exist for hearing improvement in a number of autoimmune diseases, as a sizable percentage of patients with AIED have a systemic autoimmune disease.[59]

CHALLENGES IN DETERMINING EFFICACY OF BIOLOGICS IN IMMUNE-MEDIATED SENSORINEURAL HEARING LOSS

One of the largest issues in determining efficacy of biologics for immune-mediated hearing loss is the reality that these are rare diseases with poor phenotypic features that make definitive diagnosis challenging and assessment of treatment effect similarly difficult. Most forms of immune-mediated hearing loss can likely be classified as orphan diseases, but have not, likely based on the absence of a durable biomarker that can measure the duration of active disease. Orphan disease status requires less than 200,000 afflicted patients, and provides pharmaceutical companies financial incentives to produce drugs under the orphan drug act for these rare diseases, because otherwise the paucity of afflicted patients would not make it financially feasible to proceed.[60] Moreover, given the fluctuating, chronic disease in both AIED and Meniere's disease, providing a measure of disease duration is imprecise and involves speculation of probability rather than an accurate calculation. In addition, measuring treatment efficacy also poses challenges in rare disorders in which the disease waxes and wanes. If investigators are able to provide a clear definition of disease incidence, prevalence, and duration, and establish measures of efficacy that is accepted by regulatory agencies, then approval for biologics for immune-mediated hearing loss is likely to occur.

DISCLOSURE

Dr Vambutas has previously served on the scientific advisory board of Sobi Pharmaceuticals and presently receives drug and placebo for an active clinical trial.

REFERENCES

1. McCabe BF. Autoimmune sensorineural hearing loss. Ann Otol Rhinol Laryngol 1979;88:585–9.

2. Vambutas A, Lesser M, Mullooly V, et al. Early efficacy trial of anakinra in corticosteroid-resistant autoimmune inner ear disease. J Clin Invest 2014;124(9):4115–22.
3. Broughton SS, Meyerhoff WE, Cohen SB. Immune mediated inner ear disease: 10-year experience. Semin Arthritis Rheum 2004;34:544–8.
4. Hughes GB, Barna BP, Kinney SE, et al. Clinical diagnosis of immune inner-ear disease. Laryngoscope 1988;98:251–3.
5. Frejo L, Soto-Varela A, Santos-Perez S, et al. Clinical subgroups in bilateral Meniere disease. Front Neurol 2016;7:182.
6. Hietikko E, Sorri M, Männikkö M, et al. Higher prevalence of autoimmune diseases and longer spells of vertigo in patients affected with familial Meniere's disease: a clinical comparison of familial and sporadic Meniere's disease. Am J Audiol 2014;23(2):232–7.
7. Caorsi R, Federici S, Gattorno M. Biologic drugs in autoinflammatory syndromes. Autoimmun Rev 2012;12(1):81–6.
8. Kastner DL, Aksentijevich I, Goldbach-Mansky R. Autoinflammatory disease reloaded: a clinical perspective. Cell 2010;140(6):784–90.
9. Muckle TJ. The 'Muckle-Wells' syndrome. Br J Dermatol 1979;100(1):87–92.
10. Agostini L, Martinon F, Burns K, et al. NALP3 forms an IL-1beta-processing inflammasome with increased activity in Muckle-Wells autoinflammatory disorder. Immunity 2004;20(3):319–25.
11. Tayer-Shifman OE, Ilan O, Tovi H, et al. Cogan's syndrome–clinical guidelines and novel therapeutic approaches. Clin Rev Allergy Immunol 2014;47(1):65–72.
12. Vambutas A, Pathak S. AAO: autoimmune and autoinflammatory (disease) in otology: what is new in immune-mediated hearing loss. Laryngoscope Investig Otolaryngol 2016;1(5):110–5.
13. Bloch DB, San Martin JE, Rauch SD, et al. Serum antibodies to heat shock protein 70 in sensorineural hearing loss. Arch Otolaryngol Head Neck Surg 1995;121(10):1167–71.
14. Trune DR, Kempton JB, Mitchell CR, et al. Failure of elevated heat shock protein 70 antibodies to alter cochlear function in mice. Hear Res 1998;116:65–70.
15. Tebo AE, Szankasi P, Hillman TA, et al. Antibody reactivity to heat shock protein 70 and inner ear-specific proteins in patients with idiopathic sensorineural hearing loss. Clin Exp Immunol 2006;146(3):427–32.
16. Baek MJ, Park HM, Johnson JM, et al. Increased frequencies of cochlin-specific T cells in patients with autoimmune sensorineural hearing loss. J Immunol 2006;177(6):4203–10.
17. Pathak S, Hatam LJ, Bonagura V, et al. Innate immune recognition of molds and homology to the inner ear protein, cochlin, in patients with autoimmune inner ear disease. J Clin Immunol 2013;33(7):1204–15.
18. Pathak S, Hatam LJ, Bonagura V, et al. Innate immune recognition of molds and homology to the inner ear protein, cochlin, in patients with autoimmune inner ear disease. J Clin Immunol 2013;33(7):1204–15.
19. Wilson WR, Byl FM, Laird N. The efficacy of steroids in the treatment of idiopathic sudden hearing loss. A double-blind clinical study. Arch Otolaryngol 1980;106(12):772–6.
20. Moskowitz D, Lee KJ, Smith HW. Steroid use in idiopathic sudden sensorineural hearing loss. Laryngoscope 1984;94(5 Pt 1):664–6.
21. Mattox DE, Simmons FB. Natural history of sudden sensorineural hearing loss. Ann Otol Rhinol Laryngol 1977;86(4 Pt 1):463–80.

22. Chen CY, Halpin C, Rauch SD. Oral steroid treatment of sudden sensorineural hearing loss: a ten year retrospective analysis. Otol Neurotol 2003;24(5):728–33.
23. Rauch SD, Halpin CF, Antonelli PJ, et al. Oral vs intratympanic corticosteroid therapy for idiopathic sudden sensorineural hearing loss: a randomized trial. JAMA 2011;305(20):2071–9.
24. Battaglia A, Burchette R, Cueva R. Combination therapy (intratympanic dexamethasone + high-dose prednisone taper) for the treatment of idiopathic sudden sensorineural hearing loss. Otol Neurotol 2008;29(4):453–60.
25. Battaglia A, Lualhati A, Lin H, et al. A prospective, multi-centered study of the treatment of idiopathic sudden sensorineural hearing loss with combination therapy versus high-dose prednisone alone: a 139 patient follow-up. Otol Neurotol 2014;35(6):1091–8.
26. Niparko JK, Wang NY, Rauch SD, et al. Serial audiometry in a clinical trial of AIED treatment. Otol Neurotol 2005;26(5):908–17.
27. Lorenz RR, Solares CA, Williams P, et al. Interferon-gamma production to inner ear antigens by T cells from patients with autoimmune sensorineural hearing loss. J Neuroimmunol 2002;130(1–2):173–8.
28. Fukushima K, Kasai N, Ueki Y, et al. A gene for fluctuating, progressive autosomal dominant nonsyndromic hearing loss, DFNA16, maps to chromosome 2q23-24.3. Am J Hum Genet 1999;65(1):141–50.
29. Hillman TM, Arriaga MA, Chen DA. Intratympanic steroids: do they acutely improve hearing in cases of cochlear hydrops? Laryngoscope 2003;113(11): 1903–7.
30. Leng Y, Liu B, Zhou R, et al. Repeated courses of intratympanic dexamethasone injection are effective for intractable Meniere's disease. Acta Otolaryngol 2017; 137(2):154–60.
31. Svrakic M, Pathak S, Goldofsky E, et al. Diagnostic and prognostic utility of measuring tumor necrosis factor in the peripheral circulation of patients with immune-mediated sensorineural hearing loss. Arch Otolaryngol Head Neck Surg 2012;138(11):1052–8.
32. Liu D, Ahmet A, Ward L, et al. A practical guide to the monitoring and management of the complications of systemic corticosteroid therapy. Allergy Asthma Clin Immunol 2013;9(1):30.
33. Matteson EL, Choi HK, Poe DS, et al. Etanercept therapy for immune-mediated cochleovestibular disorders: a multicenter, open-label, pilot study. Arthritis Rheum 2005;53:337–42.
34. Cohen S, Shoup A, Weisman MH, et al. Etanercept treatment for autoimmune inner ear disease: results of a pilot placebo-controlled study. Otol Neurotol 2005; 26(5):903–7.
35. Satoh H, Firestein GS, Billings PB, et al. Tumor necrosis factor-alpha, an initiator, and etanercept, an inhibitor of cochlear inflammation. Laryngoscope 2002; 112(9):1627–34.
36. Van Wijk F, Staecker H, Keithley E, et al. Local perfusion of the tumor necrosis factor alpha blocker infliximab to the inner ear improves autoimmune neurosensory hearing loss. Audiol Neurootol 2006;11(6):357–65.
37. Derebery MJ, Staecker H, Keithley E, et al. An open label study to evaluate the safety and efficacy of intratympanic golimumab therapy in patients with autoimmune inner ear disease. Otol Neurotol 2014;35(9):1515–21.
38. Haynes BF, Pikus A, Kaiser-Kupfer M, et al. Successful treatment of sudden hearing loss in Cogan's syndrome with corticosteroids. Arthritis Rheum 1981;24(3): 501–3.

39. Ghadban R, Couret M, Zenone T. Efficacy of infliximab in Cogan's syndrome. J Rheumatol 2008;35(12):2456–8.
40. Mirault T, Launay D, Cuisset L, et al. Recovery from deafness in a patient with Muckle-Wells syndrome treated with anakinra. Arthritis Rheum 2006;54(5): 1697–700.
41. Kuemmerle-Deschner JB, Koitschev A, Tyrrell PN, et al. Early detection of sensorineural hearing loss in Muckle-Wells-syndrome. Pediatr Rheumatol Online J 2015;13(1):43.
42. Vambutas A, DeVoti J, Goldofsky E, et al. Alternate splicing of interleukin-1 receptor type II (IL1R2) in vitro correlates with clinical glucocorticoid responsiveness in patients with AIED. PLoS One 2009;4(4):e5293.
43. Pathak S, Goldofsky E, Vivas EX, et al. IL-1beta is overexpressed and aberrantly regulated in corticosteroid nonresponders with autoimmune inner ear disease. J Immunol 2011;186(3):1870–9.
44. Cipriani P, Ruscitti P, Carubbi F, et al. Methotrexate: an old new drug in autoimmune disease. Expert Rev Clin Immunol 2014;10(11):1519–30.
45. Harris JP, Weisman MH, Derebery JM, et al. Treatment of corticosteroid-responsive autoimmune inner ear disease with methotrexate: a randomized controlled trial. JAMA 2003;290(14):1875–83.
46. Kuriya B, Arkema EV, Bykerk VP, et al. Efficacy of initial methotrexate monotherapy versus combination therapy with a biological agent in early rheumatoid arthritis: a meta-analysis of clinical and radiographic remission. Ann Rheum Dis 2010;69(7):1298–304.
47. Ma C, Billings P, Harris JP, et al. Characterization of an experimentally induced inner ear immune response. Laryngoscope 2000;110(3 Pt 1):451–6.
48. Barkdull GC, Hondarrague Y, Meyer T, et al. AM-111 reduces hearing loss in a guinea pig model of acute labyrinthitis. Laryngoscope 2007;117(12):2174–82.
49. Suckfuell M, Lisowska G, Domka W, et al. Efficacy and safety of AM-111 in the treatment of acute sensorineural hearing loss: a double-blind, randomized, placebo-controlled phase II study. Otol Neurotol 2014;35(8):1317–26.
50. Staecker H, Jokovic G, Karpishchenko S, et al. Efficacy and safety of AM-111 in the treatment of acute unilateral sudden deafness-a double-blind, randomized, placebo-controlled phase 3 study. Otol Neurotol 2019;40(5):584–94.
51. Nagy SE, Andersson JP, Andersson UG. Effect of mycophenolate mofetil (RS-61443) on cytokine production: inhibition of superantigen-induced cytokines. Immunopharmacology 1993;26(1):11–20.
52. Allison AC. Mechanisms of action of mycophenolate mofetil. Lupus 2005; 14(Suppl 1):s2–8.
53. Hautefort C, Loundon N, Montchilova M, et al. Mycophenolate mofetil as a treatment of steroid dependent Cogan's syndrome in childhood. Int J Pediatr Otorhinolaryngol 2009;73(10):1477–9.
54. Anderka MT, Lin AE, Abuelo DN, et al. Reviewing the evidence for mycophenolate mofetil as a new teratogen: case report and review of the literature. Am J Med Genet A 2009;149A(6):1241–8.
55. Angeli SI, Abi-Hachem RN, Vivero RJ, et al. L-N-Acetylcysteine treatment is associated with improved hearing outcome in sudden idiopathic sensorineural hearing loss. Acta Otolaryngol 2012;132(4):369–76.
56. Pathak S, Stern C, Vambutas A. N-Acetylcysteine attenuates tumor necrosis factor alpha levels in autoimmune inner ear disease patients. Immunol Res 2015; 63(1–3):236–45.

57. Chen CH, Young YH. N-acetylcysteine as a single therapy for sudden deafness. Acta Otolaryngol 2016;137(1):58–62.
58. Cohen S, Roland P, Shoup A, et al. A pilot study of rituximab in immune-mediated inner ear disease. Audiol Neurootol 2011;16(4):214–21.
59. Barna BP, Hughes GB. Autoimmunity and otologic disease: clinical and experimental aspects. Clin Lab Med 1988;8(2):385–98.
60. Aronson JK. Rare diseases and orphan drugs. Br J Clin Pharmacol 2006;61(3): 243–5.

Special Article Series: Intentionally Shaping the Future of Otolaryngology

Editor

JENNIFER A. VILLWOCK

OTOLARYNGOLOGIC CLINICS OF NORTH AMERICA

www.oto.theclinics.com

Consulting Editor
SUJANA S. CHANDRASEKHAR

August 2021 • Volume 54 • Number 4

Foreword
Building the Future We Wish to See

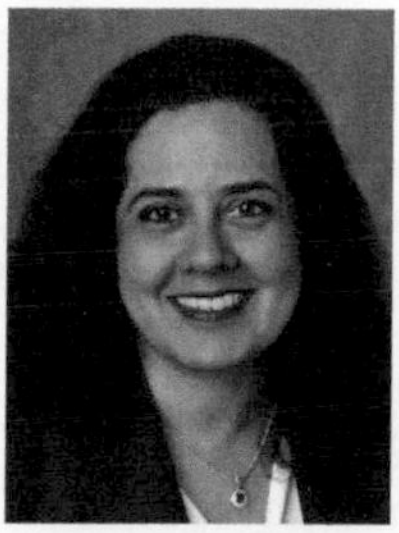

Sujana S. Chandrasekhar, MD, FACS, FAAOHNS
Consulting Editor

Dr Jennifer Villwock approached me in December of 2018 with a suggestion for an issue of *Otolaryngologic Clinics of North America* on leadership, mentorship, and professional development. As she, our then-Senior *Otolaryngologic Clinics of North America* Editor Jessica McCool, and I brainstormed as to how to craft this necessary and important series of articles so that they might reach the widest possible audience, we decided to publish them over the course of a year as a Special Article Series on Intentionally Shaping the Future of Otolaryngology, guest edited by Dr Villwock. The first two articles of the series were published in the August 2020 issue of *Otolaryngologic Clinics of North America*, and the final two articles appear in the August 2021 issue. Taken together, these 12 articles make a comprehensive treasure trove of material that is of value not just to all otolaryngologists but also to anyone who cares to see a more inclusive and fairer world.

The two Special Series articles in the current issue are "Women in Academic Medicine and Leadership" by Dr Mona M. Abaza and "Balance Versus Integration: Work-Life Considerations" by Drs Julie L. Wei and Jennifer A. Villwock. These articles explore vitally important subjects and provide an excellent conclusion to the series.

In the United States in 2004, there were four female chairs of otolaryngology (4/104 departments, 3.8%) and in 2018 there were six female chairs of otolaryngology (6/117, 5%).[1] As of December 31, 2020, the American Association of Medical Colleges reports that 4 of 86 (4.7%) US Otolaryngology departments were led by women, 3 of whom are white and 1 of whom is Asian.[2] The American Academy of Otolaryngology–Head and Neck Surgery has had only four women Presidents to date, the first of whom, Dr M. Jennifer Derebery, served in 2003-2004, and the second, Dr Gayle Woodson, served in 2014-2015. The first and only female President of the Triological Society served in 2020-2021. It is not just the highest levels of leadership that are kept from women's grasps; there are numerous barriers to getting near those positions. Even accounting

Otolaryngol Clin N Am 54 (2021) xvii–xix
https://doi.org/10.1016/j.otc.2021.05.024

for hours worked, patients seen, and academic productivity, women surgeons are promoted less, paid less, and funded less than their male counterparts.[1] Dr Abaza discusses "sticky floors," "glass ceilings," avoiding "falling off the cliff," beating the odds, missing rungs on the ladder to success, building more supportive steps, and accomplishing the future that we envision. She stresses the importance of men and women promoting the advancement of women.

Many of us came of age hearing that we should strive for work-life balance; the impetus now is for work-life integration. Balance seeks to achieve an ideal state where your work and life coexist and thrive separately; integration is about bringing work and life closer together. Drs Wei and Villwock write about burnout, well-being, wellness, gender-specific challenges for integration, and microaggressions. They provide actionable details on what to consider while starting one's career and practices to follow for emotionally healthy work-life integration. When and how to seek and use counseling, coaching, and peer support conclude this article.

The late actor Christopher Reeve, who played Superman among other characters, and sustained a complete C1-C2 vertebral injury in 1995, leaving him quadriplegic, said in 1996, "So many of our dreams at first seem impossible, then they seem improbable, and then when we summon the will, they soon become inevitable."[3] I urge the reader to take the time to read these and all 12 articles in the Special Series: Intentional Shaping the Future of Otolaryngology, guest edited by Dr Jennifer Villwock and authored by thoughtful leaders in our field. Just like Superman, we can summon the will to make these necessary changes inevitable.

Sujana S. Chandrasekhar, MD, FACS, FAAOHNS
Consulting Editor
Otolaryngologic Clinics of North America
Past President, American Academy of
Otolaryngology–Head and Neck Surgery
Secretary-Treasurer, American Otological Society
Partner, ENT & Allergy Associates, LLP
18 East 48th Street, 2nd Floor
New York, NY 10017, USA

Clinical Professor, Department of Otolaryngology–
Head and Neck Surgery
Zucker School of Medicine at
Hofstra-Northwell
Hempstead, NY, USA

Clinical Associate Professor
Department of Otolaryngology–
Head and Neck Surgery
Icahn School of Medicine at Mount Sinai
New York, NY, USA

E-mail address:
ssc@nyotology.com

Website:
http://www.ears.nyc

REFERENCES

1. Available at: https://www.enttoday.org/article/women-in-otolaryngology-do-we-belong-here/. Accessed May 8, 2021.
2. Available at: https://www.aamc.org/media/9066/download. Accessed May 8, 2021.
3. Available at: http://www.chrisreevehomepage.com/sp-dnc1996.html. Accessed May 8, 2021.

Preface
From Crisis to Change

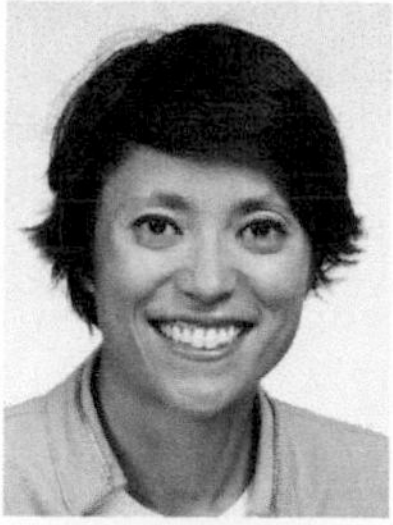

Jennifer A. Villwock, MD
Editor

The year 2020 will likely be remembered as a year of issues, many of which have been simmering under societal radar for quite some time. While the severe acute respiratory syndrome coronavirus 2 virus is the most salient example, certainly issues of systemic racism, inequities embedded in our culture, and mental wellness, or lack thereof, have touched us all as well.

It is important to remember that problems can also be invitations to not only finally acknowledge the issues but also creatively find solutions. A few short years ago, a day of "Zoom"-ing into critical meetings and seeing patients via telehealth while managing a child's remote education would have been a laughable pipedream/nightmare. Now, not only is this often the norm but also these are aspects many of us may continue to use longitudinally.

In Dr Abaza's article "Women in Academic Medicine and Leadership," she describes not only the unique issues facing women otolaryngologists in academia but also ways in which our community can provide better support. Some of these ways may be initially unfamiliar, uncomfortable, or seemingly logistically prohibitive. However, we have seen in the past year that where there is a will, there is a way. There is no better time than now to be creative, champion change, and do the work.

Dr Wei details wellness consideration for otolaryngologists in her article "Balance Versus Integration: Work-Life Considerations". She articulates the intent behind the buzzwords of "work-life balance" versus "work-life integration." Dr Wei also provides insight and information regarding unique challenges facing women, including under-discussed but critical topics like delayed childbearing and fertility, and methods for facilitating wellness at an individual and systems level.

Otolaryngol Clin N Am 54 (2021) xxi–xxii
https://doi.org/10.1016/j.otc.2021.05.023

I hope that you will find these articles informative and a starting point for continued innovation in how we can all better support each other.

Jennifer A. Villwock, MD
Department of Otolaryngology, Head and Neck Surgery
University of Kansas Medical Center
3901 Rainbow Boulevard, MS 3010
Kansas City, KS 66160, USA

E-mail address:
jvillwock@kumc.edu

Women in Academic Medicine and Leadership

Mona M. Abaza, MD, MS*

KEYWORDS

• Leadership • Women • Academics • Bias • Development

KEY POINTS

- Understanding the barriers and bias that inhibit women rising in Otolaryngology leadership is a first step to change it.
- Development and support of women by each other and current male leaders are needed to change the metrics.
- Understanding the current roles and history of women in Academic medicine and Otolaryngology are key to improving future leadership opportunities.

INTRODUCTION

Why do so many "catchy phrases" exist for describing women's leadership roles and issues? From leaky pipelines, to sticky floors, to glass ceilings and cliffs, and missing rung ladders, the language around the discussions in this area demonstrates visually the longstanding challenges and the biases faced in this area. Although these challenges are seen in many areas, less than 5% of Fortune 500 CEOs are women, they are amplified in hierarchical fields like medicine. Even when compared with other science, technology, engineering, and mathematics (STEM) fields, medicine does not fare well,[1] with surgical fields lagging even farther behind despite women scoring higher than men on numerous leadership skills.[2] Women were rated higher in 84% of leadership capacities evaluated, at all ages, despite rating themselves lower. Other diversity issues, such as race and gender identity, although not the focus of this article, compound the issues for many in our field. There are many more challenges in this area than can be covered in one article, but it will touch on a few themes and provide some concrete ideas to move forward for both those trying to advance and those helping them advance.

OUR PIPELINE

Women became the majority of entering students in college in the 1970s. STEM field degrees, although increasing by more than 55%, still only represent 32% of total

Department of Otolaryngology/Head and Neck Surgery, University of Colorado School of Medicine, 12631 East 17th Avenue, Room 3000, Aurora, CO 80045, USA
* Corresponding author:
E-mail address: Mona.abaza@cuanschutz.edu

Otolaryngol Clin N Am 54 (2021) 815–821
https://doi.org/10.1016/j.otc.2021.05.006 oto.theclinics.com
0030-6665/21/

degrees per the Educational Department statistics. Medicine has done better, with women incoming medical students representing 51.6% of their classes in 2020 and 45.6% of residents overall.[3] However, in Otolaryngology, the percentages are much lower. Although 35.8% of our current residents are women, only 13.5% of practicing Otolaryngologists are.[4] Academic medicine does worse. Only 19% of full professors are women. In 2019, only 5 women were chairs, a number too small to calculate a percentage.[3] Although it has been argued that more time is what is needed, these numbers have remained stagnant or dropped over the last 2 decades, despite the great strides toward equality at the start of the medical continuum.[4] The pipeline still leaks.

Patching Holes

Gender harassment and discrimination are significant causes of women's departure from academics. When they choose to stay, it limits their advancement. To those who would say that these concerns are a relic of times past, consider that in 2018, 40% of female medical students reported sexual harassment[1] and fears of retaliation and reprisal. Even more alarming are studies demonstrating that harassment and the disproportionate expectations for women did not correlate with intent to leave and only mildly adversely impacted job satisfaction,[5] indicating that women may accept these events as simply part of the culture. This is not acceptable. Clear leadership and reporting pathways, known and followed on all levels, and clear repercussions with violations are needed.

Implicit biases also exist in abundance. A recent report on women in surgical leadership roles stated, "increasing number of academic departments of surgery have realized that women can be inspiring and capable leaders," implying a new finding.[6] Many diversity best practices can help recruit, retain, and adequately support burgeoning leaders. Preagreed upon selection criteria that consider job skill needs can create an environment for a holistic review and a more diverse pool. Gender bias from even the name on resumes[7] and letters of recommendations[8] can be corrected by blinding them. It is also important to note that it takes several Under represented minorities (URMs) present to have an impact on a group process.[9] Although this may be difficult in smaller departments, a designated diversity representative (not just a person of a different gender or race, but a trained diversity representative) on every search committee can patch more holes.

STICKY FLOORS (OR WHAT IS LEADERSHIP?)

Traditional leadership is typically seen as the titles assigned to those more senior in an organization. However, *Forbes* describes it as having nothing to do with your title, management experience, or other typical "skills." Great leadership, the ability to empower and influence others to turn a vision into reality, is defined by its efficacy. This evolving picture of leadership as a "social influence" brings up the issues about what society views as leader qualities (more often masculine) and what might actually be more successful. Emphasizing and developing the characteristics that are needed and often used by women, versus the more traditionally masculine styles we are used to seeing, can lead to more opportunities. Chamorro-Premuzic and Gallop[10] theorized that it may not be that we lack competent women to lead but that there are too few obstacles for less competent men. The floor remains sticky.

Unsticking Feet (Yours and Others)?

Changing what is seen as valuable starts with understanding societal and our personal biases. Women are often placed in the double bind of trying to simultaneously conform to typical leadership and gender norms, which can be exact opposites. For example, being aggressive (a positive male leadership characteristic) in a woman is viewed as the "B word" (a female gender-negative characteristic).[11] Uniform implicit bias training, at a minimum for those on committees making selections, ideally for all, is a way to start culture change. Male leaders engaging new paradigms of leadership skills that normalize more traditional female characteristics linked with success,[11] such empowering belief change not just performance metrics, modeling empathy and humility, and providing more coaching, will help. There are also "expectations that women will engage in more altruistic organizational citizenship behaviors or be penalized."[5] Those institutional missions' areas are often not adequately financially incentivized, such as unfunded educational initiatives, leading to further gender disparities.

Gender biases, both organizational and personal, have measurable effects on organizational satisfaction and retention. Devaluation of women, through a lack of acknowledgment and financial inequity, is a significant contribution.[5] In a 2019 survey, women in academic otolaryngology make less than 80% of their male counterparts salaries,[3] among the worst of all specialties. Although it could be argued that women need to advocate more for themselves; even when they ask, they do not get it and can face additional consequences. In the aptly named "Social incentives for gender differences in the propensity to initiate negotiations: **sometimes it does hurt to ask**" (emphasis added by author), male evaluators often penalized women for initiating salary negotiations.[12] It is critical that the impetus of correcting this disparity not be placed on the one being undervalued. The Association of American Medical Colleges (AAMC) gender equity project has many resources for departments and institutions to make progress in this area. Lack of acknowledgment of efforts extends beyond finances. Local and national awards, panel representation, article authorship acceptance rates, journal editorial boards, and grant funding have all been found to show gender inequities.[13,14] Requirements that panels, nominating, program, and award committees be diverse are early steps. Double-blinded journal article reviews, done in many other fields, may be a step worth considering. In addition, meaningful change at the department, institutional, and national level is needed to combat these biases.

Women can work to unstick their feet and others. When women accept that they are "stuck" through self-silencing their ambition and limiting their self-aspirations, it makes it worse. Men will apply for a job when they have only a few of listed requirements and women will often not even if they have all the listed requirements, not putting themselves in line for opportunities and skill development needed to advance. Finding a personal "board of directors," a group of friends and colleagues (men or women, preferably both), or a coach to run opportunities past, can help. Developing the skills to feel confident takes real work and time. Leadership development courses to support and practice the skills that are less "natural" to women are important. Although many exist, such as Executive Leadership in Academic Medicine, AAMC early and late career courses, and individual institutional offerings, the need is often greater than the availability. More local programs, at the institutional, regional, or specialty level need to be created by tapping those who have had experienced the larger national programs and supporting the efforts needed to put them on.

GLASS CEILINGS AND OTHER HIDDEN OBSTACLES

Although glass ceilings are seen everywhere, the hierarchy of academic medicine can make advancement challenges more invisible. From a disproportionate share of domestic duties like child and elder care that can impact traditional timed promotion pathways to the unrecognized value of "community work" done within departments, women often face choices around decisions affecting advancement that their male counterparts do not. Two-career families where moving a spouse is not possible more commonly affects women, limiting career mobility. Although this is changing, generational differences are not the only obstacles. Even how a woman communicated may be a barrier, with women's voices being considered "shrill," to facing constant interruptions to conforming while also being penalized for more "passive" feminine communication styles. It can be harder for women to simply be heard, let alone be perceived as an effective leader.[15]

Burnout data even before COVID indicated that women were at a higher risk for suicide and burnout. COVID has disproportionately negatively impacted the academic productivity of women, with long-term effects on future promotions, grants, and so forth. The ceiling is still glass.

Breaking Through the Glass

Traditional academic promotion and advancement have long been based on the achievement of milestones in the clinical, research, and educational realms. However, what if this does not represent the skillset needed among leaders in the ever-increasingly complex academic medicine system? Caring for patients is the center of our profession, and women have demonstrated better outcomes in primary care mortality[16] and surgical complications,[17] but it is not the most valuated aspect in promotion. Mona Hanna-Attisha said it well during the 2020 presentation of the Vilcek-Gold Humanism Award at the AAMC 2020 Learn Serve Lead conference, "No one has even been promoted to tenure for exceptional patient care alone." Specific attention to women in any academic pathway is needed to help those trying to advance. This can include creating more academic advancement opportunities in less typical areas, such as community advocacy and patient care leaders. Providing direct support, not just for women, in the area of childcare and family support may also help more atypical leadership pathways and skills to develop. Creating a culture whereby nontraditional endeavors receive similar weight as more traditional metrics will be critical to an engage a diverse otolaryngology work force for the future.[18]

Communication does have documented gender differences. Women must be aware of hesitant speech, pitch elevation, and other issues that can impact how they are viewed when they need to be heard and how they can be more effective communicators.[15] From practicing critical communications before having them, to having others listen to them beforehand, there are many ways to work on this. In addition, others need to be better listeners. Every woman can describe a meeting where they stated an idea that was ignored. Nevertheless, 10 minutes later, the same idea is repeated by male colleague and greeted with enthusiasm and support. Women need to amplify each other's voices, as do our male colleagues. This can be as simple as repeating your female colleagues' names in reference to their contributions and expertise when it seems to go unnoticed or is attributed to someone else.

The long-standing absence of succession planning in academic medicine, although not true for every department or school, needs to be mentioned as a part of the difficulty in advancing. The "dying at your desk" attitude is present everywhere in medicine. It is not possible to make significant change in national leadership numbers if there is no room to advance. A unique idea is to set term limits in an academic medicine leadership role.[19] In addition to diversifying leadership more quickly, it could lead to more opportunities for new roles in our departments for those in the latter parts of their career.

FALLING OFF A CLIFF (SET UP TO FAIL)

Even when women make it through the ceiling, they are often surprised to find themselves on a glass cliff (high-risk role with little opportunity to succeed) with no support.

"We gave a woman a chance, but she failed" becomes an intentionally self-fulfilling prophecy. Described as "male privilege," many academic environments have a culture where informal discussions and events ("the meeting before the meeting") take place in situations in which women are not always included. This limits access to the information needed to be successful.[5] The hierarchal nature of medicine and the limited numbers of women have also created a situation where men are the "gatekeepers" of leadership positions, making their perceptions the dominate ones. In addition, women are pressured to hire men under them to "balance" the team.[5]

The "queen-bee" effect (being the only woman leader and used as an example that there is "enough" representation) can cause resentment by others and correlates with increased turnover and decreased job satisfaction.[5] This combined with the burden of tokenism (the challenge of being the sole representative of your gender or race) for an organization contributes to women being viewed as less supportive of each other's success and sometimes actually being less supportive.[5] Two-career families are more common with women leaders, leading to more challenges regarding the social support roles that spouses are expected to perform, which are more noticeable the higher the position. The cliff is glass and slippery.

Beating the odds (safety ropes needed)

Having a clear understanding of your personal goals, vision, and what the job actually entails is important to know before you take a job. Taking a position just for a title, especially if it is not aligned with your goals, is unlikely to result in success and fulfillment. Assuming a role without the needed support, financial, support staff, time, technology, to be successful is also a sure way to fail. Ask for it up front. You are less likely to get it later on.

Also, women can learn from male colleagues. Men more often view a career setback as just that, not a personal determination of their worth. Adopting a bit more of the "it's just business" attitude can help women to stop limiting themselves. Keep trying even when you do not want to. Find time to nurture yourself and find friends to help you. No failure is final; it will not be the last one you have. Support each other, those with you, and those below and above you. As Dennis Waitley said, "Success is not pie with a limited number of pieces." Building opportunities for others should increase opportunities for all, so all should speak out when it does not.

WHY CAN'T I GET UP THIS LADDER? (MISSING RUNGS)

Even with all the self-determination and self-preparation, it is still tougher for women to climb up the leadership structure. The rungs are further apart than many can reach, and even when they can, it can get pretty tiring halfway up. Common missing rungs often cited are inadequate mentoring and sponsorship. Typical opportunities for informal mentoring, late meetings, drinks after events, panels and course speaker invitations, and other activities may leave women excluded. Even more formal opportunities have their own challenges. Unfortunately, a repercussion of the #MeToo movement has made some men fearful that mentoring will place them in jeopardy.

Women are often overmentored and undersponsored.[20] Although many men feel they provide supportive advice to women (mentoring), few women have good sponsorship. It is one thing to tell the story of how you got to the position you have; it is another to specifically put someone in place to succeed you. As mentioned, women's careers are also less likely to follow a "traditional" path. Understanding that your mentee may not only be unable, but may not want, to follow your exact path is important for mentors to realize when offering advice. The rungs are missing.

BUILDING MORE SUPPORTIVE STEPS

Improving networking opportunities and understanding the "hidden curriculum" of leadership (such as the "meeting before the meeting") are important. Although women need to network independently, and many opportunities like the Women in Otolaryngology Section events and other specialty society women's section exist for that, it is not enough on its own. It cannot be underestimated how much need there is for those actually in power now to directly value and seek women's contributions. The "He for She" movement and true sponsorship to promote women to power positions are critically needed at every level. Nominating a woman for a position, an award, or a new opportunity, even when she does not ask (because she will not) is important but understanding if it is part of her goals is even more so.

Understanding, developing, and engaging in newer paradigms for successful mentoring programs is needed for the future Otolaryngology. For many of the older among us, mentoring meant you found someone you wanted to be and then attempted to emulate them. The complex changes and compartmentalization of academic medicine make this a less successful strategy today and, as noted, even less so for women. Active mentoring is more than creating a copy of your career but is aiding someone to create one you had not imagined. Mentees are not passive receptacles of knowledge but active partners in creating a supportive future that fits their goals and personal vision.

THE FUTURE

Elizabeth Blackwell became the first woman doctor in 1859, and today more than 50% of entering medical students are women. It is long past time for an equal place in academic medicine leadership. Otolaryngology lags behind other fields in metrics in this area, but the smaller size and closeness of our field have allowed us to make many bold steps in education and patient care. It can help us here as well. Women in our field have to support themselves with clearly articulated goals and aspirations and serve as role models to the next generation. However, help is also needed. Our departments and institutions need to create new opportunities and level the playing field. Our male colleagues and leaders need to be active in support and open to change. Together we can clean our floors, shatter our ceiling and cliffs, and create well-made ladders for women and all URMs in Otolaryngology to climb. It will make all of Otolaryngology better for all of us.

CLINICS CARE POINTS

- Women continue to not be represented adequately in academic otolaryngology advancement and leadership roles over many decades.
- Institutions and departments need to make definitive efforts to change this and support their current students, residents, and fellows.
- Bias mitigation processes and other equity practices should be applied to all institutions and departments to affect change.

DISCLOSURES

Dr Abaza serves as President of the Otolaryngology Women's Leadership Society (OtoWLS) and as a board member of the Accreditation Council of Graduate Medical Education (ACGME). Received Board Grant from Josiah Macy Jr. Foundation.

REFERENCES

1. National Academies of Sciences. Engineering, and Medicine. In: Sexual harassment of women: climate, culture, and consequences in academic sciences, engineering, and medicine. Washington, DC: The National Academies Press; 2018. https://doi.org/10.17226/24994. Available at:.
2. Zenger J, Folkman J. Research: women score higher than men in most leadership skills. Harvard Business Review. Available at: https://hbr.org/2019/06/research-women-score-higher-than-men-in-most-leadership-skills. Accessed June 25, 2019.
3. Association of American Medical Colleges. 2019. Washington, DC. Available at:https://www.aamc.org/data-reports/data/2018-2019-state women-academic-medicine-exploring-pathways-equity. Accessed March 11, 2020.
4. O'Connell Ferster AP, Hu A. Women in otolaryngology. Otolaryngol Head Neck Surg 2017;157(2):173–4.
5. Diehl AB, Stephenson AL, Dzubinski LM, et al. Measuring the invisible: development and multi-industry validation of the gender bias scale for women leaders. Hum Res Dev Q 2020;31:249–80.
6. Pories SE, Turner PL, Greenburg CC, et al. Leadership in American surgery; women are rising to the top. Ann Surg 2019;269(2):199–205.
7. Moss-Racusin CA, Dovidio JF, Brescoll VL, et al. Faculty's subtle gender biases favor male students. Proc Natl Acad Sci 2012;2012:201211286.
8. Turrentine FE, Dreisbach CN, St Ivany AR, et al. Influence of gender on surgical residency applicants' recommendation letters. J Am Coll Surg 2019;228(4): 356–65.e3.
9. Woolley AW, Chabris CF, Pentland A, et al. Evidence for a collective intelligence factor in the performance of human groups Science 2010.
10. Chamorro-Premuzic, T. and Gallop, C. 7 leadership lessons men can learn from women. Harv Business Rev, 2020.
11. Kubu CS. Who does she think she is? Women, leadership and the 'B' (ias) word. Clin Neuropysch 2018;32(2):235–51.
12. Organizational behavior and human decision processes 103; 2007:84-103.
13. Hankivsky O, Springer KW, Hunting G. Beyond sex and gender difference in funding and reporting of health research. Res Integr Peer Rev 2018;3:6.
14. Lundine J, Bourgeault IL, Clark J, et al. The gendered system of academic publishing. Lancet 2018;391:1754–6.
15. Cundiff JL, Vescio TK. Gender stereotypes influence how people explain gender disparities in the workplace. Sex Roles 2016;75:126–38.
16. Tsugawa Y, Jena AB, Figueroa JF, et al. Comparison of hospital mortality and readmission rates for Medicare patients treated by male vs female physicians. JAMA Intern Med 2017;177(2):206–13.
17. Wallis C, Rav i B, Coburn N, et al. Comparison of postoperative outcomes among patients treated by male and female surgeons: a population based matched cohort study. BMJ 2017;359:j4366.
18. Boysen PG 2nd, Daste L, Northern T. Multigenerational challenges and the future of graduate medical education. Ochsner J 2016;16(1):101–7.
19. Austin JP. Is academic medicine ready for term limits? Acad Med 2020;95(2): 180–3.
20. Ibarra H. A lack of sponsorship is keeping women from advancing into leadership. 2019. Harvard Business Review. Available at: https://hbr.org/2019/08/a-lack-of-sponsorship-is-keeping-women-from-advancing-into-leadership. Accessed March 11, 2020.

Balance Versus Integration

Work-Life Considerations

Julie L. Wei, MD[a,*], Jennifer A. Villwock, MD[b]

KEYWORDS

• Work-life integration • Work-life balance • Well-being • Engagement
• Micropractices • Microaggression

KEY POINTS

- Work-life integration reflects the synergy needed between professional and personal lives only achievable by creating strategies that optimize holistic self-care and efficiencies in both.
- There are gender-specific differences and various factors that increase challenges to achieve work-life integration. Awareness and intentional strategies can be used to mitigate challenges.
- Micropractices can increase work-life integration: including creating routines for gratitude, self-compassion, time management, healthy nutrition, exercise, outsourcing, finding support, and setting realistic expectations.
- Normalizing individual and relationship counseling and use of mental health support are critical to enhance work-life integration, minimize burnout, and optimize well-being.
- Formal and informal peer support are necessary to minimize second-victim effects from the cumulative impact of the acute and chronic stress inherent to the practice of medicine and surgery.

INTRODUCTION

Health care culture and attitudes have lagged behind other industries on the now highly visible topic of burnout. This topic includes conversations on the associated topics of wellness, well-being, and strategies to achieve work-life balance and/or work-life integration. Much research and data have validated why employee burnout must be addressed; the psychological and physical issues of burned-out employees cost an estimated $125 billion to $190 billion a year in US health care spending.[1] Burnout in

[a] Pediatric Otolaryngology/Audiology, GME Wellbeing Initiatives, Nemours Children's Hospital, Otolaryngology Education, Otolaryngology Head Neck Surgery, University of Central Florida College of Medicine, 6535 Nemours Parkway, Orlando, FL 32827, USA; [b] Department of Otolaryngology–Head Neck Surgery, University of Kansas Medical Center, 3901 Rainbow Boulevard, Kansas City, KS 66160, USA

* Corresponding author. Division Otolaryngology, 6535 Nemours Parkway, Orlando, FL 32827.
E-mail address: Julie.Wei@Nemours.Org
Twitter: @drjuliewei (J.L.W.)

Otolaryngol Clin N Am 54 (2021) 823–837
https://doi.org/10.1016/j.otc.2021.05.007
0030-6665/21/

physicians and health care professionals can have additional, and profound, impacts on society at large and health care organizations. Beyond decreased productivity and costs associated with turnover, physician wellness is vital to the delivery of high-quality care. For example, burnout has been associated with increased medical errors and less compassionate care in numerous studies.[2] Mandates to improve care and outcomes and achieve the goal of zero harm cannot be successful if physician wellness is not simultaneously prioritized. It has been hypothesized that physician wellness is a missing quality indicator and optimization of patient-centered care cannot occur without it.[3]

Although burnout and achieving individual and system well-being is beyond the scope of this article and is addressed elsewhere,[4] this article explores considerations that can support optimal work-life integration or balance. Definitions of terms commonly used when discussing physician realities of burnout, well-being, and the challenges of managing work and life are outlined next.

Burnout

A syndrome conceptualized as a result of chronic workplace stress that has not been successfully managed. It is characterized by 3 dimensions[5]:

1. Feeling of energy depletion or exhaustion
2. Increased mental distance from one's job, or feeling of negativism or cynicism related to one's job
3. Reduced professional efficacy

Of note, burnout refers specifically to phenomena in the occupational context and should not be applied to describe experiences in other areas of life.

Wellness

The optimal state of health of individuals and groups with 2 focal concerns: (1) the realization of the fullest potential of an individual physically, psychologically, socially, spiritually, and economically; and (2) the fulfillment of one's role expectations in the family, community, place of worship, workplace, and other settings.[6]

Well-being

The state or experience of being happy, healthy, or prosperous. This state includes good mental health, high life satisfaction, being socially connected, having a sense of meaning or purpose, and ability to manage stress.[7]

Balance

Noun: physical equilibrium; stability; aesthetically pleasing integration of elements; mental and emotional steadiness.

Verb: to poise or arrange in, or as if in, balance; to bring into harmony or proportion; to bring to a state or position of balance.[8]

Integration

Noun: the act or instance of combining into an integral whole; behavior, as of an individual that is in harmony with the environment

Verb: to bring together or incorporate parts into a whole; to unite or combine; to give, or cause to give, equal opportunity and consideration to things (eg, racial, religious, or ethnic groups).[9]

WORK-LIFE INTEGRATION VERSUS WORK-LIFE BALANCE

According to University of California Berkeley Haas School of Business, there is a difference between these 2 terms. Work-life balance evokes a binary opposition between work and life, creating a sense of competition between the 2 elements, whereas integration describes an approach that creates more synergies between all areas that define life: work, home, family, community, personal well-being, and health.[10] Ideally, all these aspects are blended into a unified whole.[11]

Throughout surgical training, the overall educational focus has been on progressive mastery in clinical decision making, surgical competence, autonomy, minimizing mistakes, and achieving independent competence to practice the subspecialty of choice. Since 2017, the Accreditation Council for Graduate Medical Education mandates that all training programs have a specific wellness program for residents and faculty, as 1 of the 6 areas of assessment to achieve accreditation.[12] The culture of well-being and how organizations function as learning environments is now a key focus for accreditation review.

After training and starting their careers, surgeons are lifelong learners and continue to master surgical procedures while acquiring additional knowledge via direct experience and required continuing medical education. For a subset of surgeons, honing teaching, research, administrative, and other educational expertise is also critical to their career development. Simultaneously, surgeons also receive day-to-day cumulative exposure to demands beyond the scheduled clinical and surgical care of patients. This exposure includes emergencies, clerical and documentation burdens, time and effort on committees, and theoretic 24-7 availability through online messaging, often with patients and their families expecting immediate responses. How to successfully navigate these demands in real time during and after clinical care and work hours is rarely taught during formal training. The consequence of these chronic imbalances lead to perpetual daily perception and experience of high degrees of stress, perception of inadequacy, physical and emotional exhaustion, lack of self-care, and psychosocial morbidity, including hopelessness, depression, and suicidality. In addition, the inner narrative for physicians and surgeons becomes one of chronic time scarcity, with no time available for anything that is not patient or medicine related. Sixty-four percent of surgeons think that their work schedule does not leave adequate time for personal and family life.[13]

The solution is not for clinicians to master more multitasking, nor is truly balancing these priorities possible. Knowing that these struggles exist, and with different frequencies and manifestations depending on the individual, how do clinicians build a healthier work-life integration? First, they must forgo the belief that there is any balance to be had. Accepting the reality of their professionally and personally integrated lives may allow them to develop new perspectives and beliefs that can create change in behavior and increase individual well-being. Focusing on self-love, self-compassion, and willingness to embrace our humanness, including limitations, is critical to holistic well-being. It is also important to note that work-life integration is often a moving target. Lack of work-life integration is not a personal failure. Physicians desire to serve their patients with energy and compassion as well as have a healthy life outside of medicine.[14] As an aptly titled article notes, "Work/Life Balance: It Is Just Plain Hard."[15]

COVID-19 AND PHYSICIAN WELLNESS

The COVID-19 (coronavirus disease 2019) pandemic has added additional dimensions to the immense stress chronically faced by physicians. The pandemic meets all the criteria for a traumatic event as defined by the *Diagnostic and Statistical Manual of*

Mental Disorders, Fifth Edition.[16] COVID-19 is outside the range of normal human experience, markedly distressing to almost anyone, and involves a perceived intense threat to life, physical integrity, intense fear, helplessness, or horror. It is not surprising that COVID-19 has exacerbated existing and accumulated mental health issues among physicians. As in prior modern epidemics, such as the 2003 severe acute respiratory syndrome (SARS) outbreak, the long-term psychological impacts that will need to be addressed to optimize physician wellness include acute stress disorder, posttraumatic stress disorder, depression, anxiety, and substance abuse.[17]

Although some of the ramifications of the pandemic have been positive, such as accelerated individual and organizational adoption of technology to support collaboration and the ability to work virtually, it has also created new daily challenges, especially for women, who typically shoulder most of the burden of household labor and are more likely to head single-parent households.[18] Examples of new challenges include trying to simultaneously work and facilitate virtual school; caring for young children, elderly, or at-risk family members[19]; and managing competing demands amid constant change and evolving public health considerations. There are also additional systems stresses that are directly experienced by individuals, such as staffing shortages.[20] In addition, political and social unrest has created profound individual stress on top of chronic work-related stress, particularly for health care professionals who belong to minoritized groups. Given uncertainty related to the pandemic, public health issues, and associated inherent risks to personal safety, creating awareness and helping physicians engage in authentic actions to optimize well-being is more critical than ever.

GENDER-SPECIFIC DIFFERENCES AND CHALLENGES AT WORK AND HOME

Gender differences in personality, communication, leadership, and performance have long been a subject of interest. Although gender differences in personality are a subject of debate, there is no clear consensus. Recent studies of the personality profiles of otolaryngology faculty and residents have shown that men and women otolaryngologists are more similar than they are different. Gender differences were subtle compared with the broad range of individual differences within each gender.[21] In another study, the same 3 factors (hours worked per week, work-home conflict in the last 3 weeks, and resolving most recent work-home conflict in favor of work) were independently associated with burnout in both women and men surgeons. For both genders, work-home conflicts are rarely resolved with personal or family priorities taking precedence over work.[22] As such, although there are stereotyped gender differences, treating each person as an individual is recommended rather than assuming that they will behave in accordance with gender norms.

However, there are noteworthy differences in expectations for different genders that can significantly affect both work-life integration and overall well-being, particularly in surgeons. Women are more likely to be in personal relationships where both partners are working.[22] They also spend more time on domestic and parenting responsibilities. Women are also significantly more likely to report conflict between their own career and that of their spouse/partner. When these conflicts occur, it was 3-fold more likely for women surgeons that the conflict was resolved in favor of their spouse.[22] It is often assumed that these gender differences are dissipating as more women enter the physician workforce. However, a 2014 study of Generation X physician-researchers found that women with children, even after controlling for professional work hours and spousal employment, spent 8.5 hours per week more on parenting or domestic activities than men.[23] Many physician-mothers report sole responsibility for most domestic tasks.[24] Traditionally held beliefs about women's role in the home and workforce remain true for a large segment of the US women surgeon population. In addition, men with spouses or domestic partners who do not work full time may not appreciate challenges faced by their women colleagues, who are more likely to be in relationships where both partners work.[23] This lack of recognition hinders the ability for the culture of medicine, and its predominantly male leadership, to appropriately support women.

The culture of the medical profession has been recognized as a key factor that might deter doctors from taking care of themselves. In a study of physicians' attitudes toward their own health, Thompson and colleagues[25] identified that general practitioners feel pressure from both their patients and colleagues to appear physically well, even when they are sick, because they believe their health is interpreted as an indicator of their medical competence. Similarly, McKevitt and colleagues[26] reported that more than 80% of the general practitioners and hospital doctors in their study worked through their illness. Their results from interviews with doctors showed that professional and organizational barriers, which reinforce one another, could contribute to reluctance to take sick leave or discuss health concerns with colleagues.[26] Moreover, Baldwin and colleagues[27] have shown that trainee doctors are adopting the same behavior that has been previously reported in older, more established doctors. When questioned about their response to hypothetical illnesses, 61% of junior doctors would go to work and wait and see if they were vomiting all night, 83% if they had blood in their urine, 76% if they had a suspected stomach ulcer, and 73% if they had severe anxiety.[27]

It is beyond the scope of this article to discuss in detail the differences between behavior, communication, and leadership styles between men and women and how gender-based stereotypes may negatively affect professional development, especially for women. Nonetheless, it is important to note the salient ways in which the continued application of antiquated gender expectations occurs to women leaders in medicine. For example, women continue to be stereotyped as expressing and showing more emotions. This stereotype reinforces biased beliefs that women are ineffective leaders. However, the data directly oppose these outdated beliefs. For example, reviews of data from the corporate world done by the Harvard Business Review highlight corporate data that show that women score higher than men in most leadership skills.[28] According to an analysis of thousands of 360-degree reviews, women outscored men on 17 of 19 capabilities that differentiate excellent leaders from average or poor ones. These capabilities included metrics such as taking initiatives, resilience, practices of self-development, drives for results, and develops others.[28] Beginning in 2016, the Harvard Business Review (HBR) has collected data on self-reported confidence levels. The greatest difference in confidence ratings between men and women was in those younger than 25 years, with confidence ratings merging at age 40 years. After 60 years of age, male confidence declines whereas female confidence increases. The consistent observation by HBR is that women make highly competent leaders according to those who work with them, but the ceiling and barriers are multifactorial.

Primary obstacles are cultural biases and unconscious bias against women. The stereotypes, and their implications, are simply not changing fast enough. Research validates that women leaders need to be warm and nice (traditional societal expectation from women) as well as competent and tough (societal expectation from men and leaders). However, women are often judged and labeled as either being too soft or too hard. Although much of the existing literature focuses on women, most, if not all, underrepresented groups face immense pressure to conform to stereotypes and cultural expectations and face penalties if they do not. Increased awareness among individuals, senior leadership, and health systems is critical to address unconscious bias toward not only gender-based discrimination but race, age, sexual orientation, and all profiles and defining characteristics of individuals. Greater understanding, appreciation, and intentional sponsorship are needed to advance those with the ability and desire to lead. This effort must be accompanied by an awareness of bias and a true desire to create positive work environments and model positive behaviors for trainees.

The American Association of Medical Colleges (AAMC) reported in 2013 an increase of full-time women faculty from 25% to 38% over the past 2 decades. However, gender disparities in leadership positions remain striking; there is a pattern of reduced representation of women by rank consistent across most departments. The proportion of women in department chair positions remains low.[29] Carr and colleagues[30] sampled full-time faculty from 24 randomly selected US medical schools on faculty perception of gender discrimination and sexual harassment. Questionnaires from 3332 full-time faculty showed that women faculty were more than 2.5 times more likely than men to perceive gender-based discrimination in the academic environment, and that those who experienced negative gender bias had similar productivity but lower career satisfaction scores than other women. Half of women faculty, but few faculty who were men, experienced some form of sexual harassment. Publications, career satisfaction, and professional confidence were not affected by sexual harassment. Self-assessed career advancement was only marginally lower for female faculty who had experienced sexual harassment.

INFERTILITY, PART-TIME WORK, AND BIAS

Risk of infertility is much higher for women than for men. Pursuing a career in medicine often means deferring marriage and having children as young women focus on completion of medical school, residency, and additional fellowship training. Although there may be formal and informal mentorship by women faculty, counseling regarding risk factors for infertility and options to circumvent these issues is not standard. If pregnancy does occur, the focus of parental leave policies at most institutions and within most practices is on its impact on individual and group productivity and not what is best for the new parent. Many women in medical academia view pregnancy and childrearing as having a net negative impact on their productivity and career trajectory.[24] Policies guiding treatment of those who become parents (eg, extended tenure timelines, individualized promotion criteria) are lacking, which likely contributes to the underrepresentation of women at all levels of medical and academic leadership.

Further examples of bias against women in medicine to consider when developing policies and strategies include:

- Punitive consequences and criticism after complications are worse for women surgeons. For example, primary care physicians decrease referrals to women surgeons, but not their male counterparts, after bad outcomes.[31]
- Lack of understanding and policies that provide substantive support for those who need intermittent or temporary leave, or desire to work part-time. This lack of understanding can be in the context of raising children, caring for ailing family members, maternity leave, or personal choice for any reason.
- Societal and cultural belief that time worked is the only metric directly proportional to worth as a physician and, by extension, that those who deviate from 100%-time effort devoted to clinical practice have wasted their training and are less valuable contributors to medicine and society.

- Lack of consistent and mandatory training on conscious and unconscious bias for all.
- Violation of workplace policy, retaliation, frank and subversive attacks, or creation of hostile work environment for women and other underrepresented groups. For example, openly joking about professional support or career development activities for women, making inappropriate comments about appearance, or joking about physiologic needs related to pregnancy or breastfeeding.

Speaking to those who have experienced any or all of these problems can be very helpful for younger trainees and faculty to get guidance and perspective on how to approach or handle experiences that can create emotional trauma and/or decrease confidence.

MICROAGGRESSION

Microaggression is a subtle form of bias that includes microassaults, microinsults, microinvalidations, and environmental aggressions that are expressions of indirect, subtle, and sometimes unintentional discrimination against members of a marginalized group that serve to maintain existing power structures.[32]

Originally coined in 1970 by a Harvard psychologist, the term initially referred to the minor but damaging humiliations and indignities experienced by African Americans.[33] The term has evolved in the years since to the description given earlier. The study of microaggressions is a nascent field and a detailed analysis of recent findings in medicine is beyond the scope of this article. Nonetheless, it is important to understand that they exist and are a common experience for women and individuals from minority backgrounds.[34] Microaggressions occur intentionally and unintentionally and can have a dramatic impact on not only their targets but the overall culture of medicine. This impact includes not only how clinicians interact with their colleagues and trainees but also the care rendered to patients. Microaggressions can generate stresses equal to or worse than overt discrimination.[35] Examples include addressing all physicians on an email by the title Doctor except the women, who are referred to by first name. Another common occurrence is patient disbelief that the woman or person of color who worked them up and explained a procedure and associated complications in detail is actually a surgeon because they do not look like physicians. Such microaggressions can also pathologize a person's authentic behavior and identity expression. Individuals should not have to sacrifice their authentic selves in order to conform to biased expectations.[32] Beyond sexism, other prominent microaggression themes in medicine are pregnancy and childcare related, having abilities underestimated, encountering sexually inappropriate comments, being relegated to mundane tasks, and feeling excluded/marginalized.[36]

Several strategies have been recommended for use when a microaggression occurs. It is critical to note that it is not the victim's responsibility to take action. Bystanders, particularly if they belong to the majority group, should also speak up. One recommended framework was described by Ganote and colleagues[37] and is remembered by the phrase "open the front door," for observe, think, feel, desire. Statements are made regarding what was observed, how the comment was thought about and interpreted, how it made (or may have made) the recipient feel, and what the desired outcome may be. For example, "When you said [microaggression], it made me think [negative thing]. I feel concerned about this because [reason], and I would like us to discuss this further so we can come to an understanding. Another framework is ACTION, for ask clarifying questions; come from curiosity, not judgment; tell what you observed in a factual manner; impact exploration (ie, discuss what the impact of the statement was); own your own thoughts and feelings around the situation; and next steps.[38] The ACTION framework may look like the following: "I am not sure that I understood what you meant when you said [microaggression]. I want to better understand; can you please explain that to me? When I hear comments like that, it makes me feel like you think [negative thing].[39]" Depending on the response, the discussion can close with action items for follow-up. If the person addressing the microaggression is not the intended victim, it may also be helpful to follow up with that individual to enquire about the person's well-being and ask whether there is anything that could be done differently or better the next time.

PRACTICES TO INCREASE WELLNESS AND WORK-LIFE INTEGRATION

Micropractices are those that can be readily integrated into daily life during pauses or events that already occur (**Box 1**). Examples of ongoing events include hand sanitizing/washing, lag time when logging in to an electronic system, wait time for the elevator or while taking stairs, and commute time. Are you well hydrated? Hungry? Are you carrying emotional remnants of the last difficult patient encounter? Are you processing difficult news? These recurring events can serve as a cue for a valuable wellness check, especially if used to name the experienced emotions.[40] Functional

Box 1
Factors to consider when starting a career for better work-life integration

- Degree of flexibility in clinical responsibilities.
- Establishment of reasonable goals and timelines for professional activities, such as scholarly work, publications, research, and teaching.
- Number of partners in practice setting, which has implication on call frequency as well as less tangible factors such as availability of mentoring and peer support.
- Financial well-being/protection:
  - Organizational contributions to retirement savings
  - Years until equal partnership if private practice
  - Salary and total compensation model/formula including:
    - Benchmarks
    - Bonuses
    - Educational support
    - Malpractice coverage
    - Short-term and long-term disability
    - Legal support
    - Availability of paid time off
    - Leave policies, including parental leave
- Formal and informal mentorship availability.
- Organization/employer awareness and commitment to equity, diversity, antiracism, inclusion, and transparent policies that facilitate an equitable and just culture.
- Presence and support for use of lactation rooms in various settings and work facilities inside clinics, hospitals, and research settings.
- Attitude of the chief, chair, and immediate supervisor on burnout and well-being, as well as that of the highest-ranking senior leaders for the organization.
- Organizational, department, and division leadership; demographics of those in leadership roles; and whether they represent the diversity workforce they represent.
  - Often simply walking the hallway of the C-suite, one can see the framed glamour shots of leaders and whether diversity is present.

MRI research has helped show the validity of this approach. Simply acknowledging and naming emotions can decrease emotional reactivity by shifting brain activity away from the amygdala to the prefrontal cortex, which can facilitate greater feelings of calm.[41] Lists of feelings are readily available online to facilitate this practice.[42]

Gratitude has long been anecdotally linked to improved well-being and now occupies a distinct niche within the self-help industry. Depending on the context, gratitude can be an emotion, an attitude, a moral virtue, a habit, a personality trait, or a coping response.[43] A core theme of gratitude is the recognition of a gift. When people are asked to compare thankfulness with other emotions, it is most commonly likened to joy and contentment.[44] A gratitude practice facilitates the ability to appreciate and savor the meaningful elements of daily existence.[43]

When health care workers were tasked with identifying 3 good things daily for 15 days, there were significant improvements from baseline in emotional exhaustion, depression symptoms, and happiness at 1, 6, and 12 months and in work-life balance at 1 and 6 months. Individuals who initially scored in the concerning range on baseline metrics experienced even greater positive effects.[45] Of note, the effect sizes of this daily gratitude practice were similar to those noted for selective serotonin reuptake inhibitors and mindfulness-based stress reduction interventions.[46,47] "Fill your tank" by recording a gratitude list, emotions and circumstances, epiphanies, and daily patient encounters or cases that brought positive experiences.

Note that gratitude is not limited to self-reflection practices. Meaningfully expressing gratitude can be therapeutic as well. Send messages of love and gratitude to your family, friends, neighbors, or anyone who has made your home or work life a better experience. For example, send surprise gifts, a card, chocolates, flowers, or other tokens to someone you care about or to a person who has made your life better in any way. Express gratitude to your leadership and colleagues, including trainees, when they have made you feel valued, respected, and heard or if they supported you during a moment of need.

Setting Realistic Expectations and Regaining Autonomy

Introspection is required for all individuals to understand and effectively communicate their priorities and goals, both in their professional and personal spheres of life. There are several baseline questions to ask. For example, what activities are engaged in most frequently? What are the most fulfilling? What is the time commitment and importance associated with each? From these questions, triage activities by order of necessity, importance, and fulfillment. Unless mowing the lawn, cleaning the house, or doing yardwork is personally fulfilling, consider engaging outside help to outsource the burden of these tasks.[23] There is much more work to be done to normalize and empower individual physicians to have autonomy to decide when, and under what circumstances, they want to adjust their schedule to make family obligations a priority.[48]

Time Management

Time is the most critical indispensable asset. Developing efficiency and effective time management is crucial for success. For example, avoid wasting time driving all over town to buy supplies that can be ordered. This time could be better spent for exercise, hobbies, sleep, meditation, or other enjoyable activities. Making a schedule and adhering to it is also crucial.[11] Review professional commitments ahead of time. Reflect on last year: where and when did you overcommit? What did you say "Yes" to that you ended up dreading? What did you agree to that you loved doing? Consider these factors when creating schedules that are doable, avoid overcommitting, and include self-care. Self-care can include simply trying something new: Pilates, ping-pong, pickleball, yoga. When possible, schedules should be created in advance and around important activities such as birthday parties, dinners, play dates, and so forth. After committing to personal and family time, activities that you or your family really want to invest in for growth and depth can be added.

Nutrition and Exercise

Even if you do not know how, or hate, cooking, have a plan to keep your body nourished with healthy food, both at work and at home. In a 2008 survey of National Health Service physicians, nearly three-quarters of physicians indicated that hospital cafeterias did not have adequate healthy options.[49] Many meal preparation and delivery options exist. The daily work and demands of a surgical career may challenge healthy hydrating and eating habits that support blood glucose homeostasis. Because female surgeons may defer family planning and pregnancy because of length of surgical residency training and additional fellowship training, awareness of impact on blood sugar regulation as related to dietary habits and routine exercise on fertility is important.[50] Harvard researchers established relationship between fertility and diet with folic acid, vitamin B_{12}, omega-3 fatty acids, and a healthy diet having positive fertility effects, whereas antioxidants, vitamin D, dairy products, soy, caffeine, and alcohol seemed to have little or no effect on fertility.[51] In addition, muscle mass decreases with age, which is especially important for women, who typically have less muscle mass than men. For this reason, developing a physical fitness routine is important for overall health and to reduce chances of musculoskeletal-related disability.

Childcare

If you have, or are considering having, children, anticipate both routine and potential unexpected childcare (eg, sick child) needs as early as possible. Parenting responsibilities contribute significantly to work-home conflicts and overall household duties. The ability to clearly plan for these needs may mitigate future frustrations. When selecting a practice, especially if a larger hospital or academic practice, on-site or flexible hour options may be available. It is also important to note that excellent childcare support occurs in many forms: spouses, nannies (live-in or otherwise), extended family, and daycare.

COUNSELING AND COACHING

Although it is possible to write the characters "I love you," traditional Chinese culture does not include speaking these words on a daily basis, except perhaps in movies and teledrama. I lost my mother to breast cancer at age 9 years, followed immediately by immigrating to the United States, without knowing any English, and with a new stepmother. We simply did not express emotions even though experiencing deep pain from loss and grief. Despite years of what, in hindsight, was depression from unprocessed grief and challenges in adolescence, I never knew counseling existed. It was never mentioned in my culture nor did I know anyone in counseling throughout high school or college after immigrating to the United States. It was not until my third year in medical school, during my psychiatry rotation, that it was strongly suggested to me after I was outwardly expressing significant signs of depression. The immense benefit I have since experienced, not just during medical school but subsequently at intervals during residency, then as a faculty, and even now, both from individual and marital counseling, is supported by the literature.

Clough and colleagues[52] conducted a systematic review of psychosocial interventions targeting occupational stress and burnout among medical doctors. Although only 12 of 23 articles reviewed included preintervention to postintervention effects, cognitive-behavioral interventions were promising and showed the strongest evidence, particularly for reducing stress. They also concluded that additional and more rigorous studies examining the benefits of psychosocial/behavioral interventions for occupational stress and burnout in physicians are needed.[52] Factors associated with burnout in trainees and faculty in both surgical and nonsurgical fields have been better studied. In a review of 47 articles published between 2009 and 2014, Amoafo and colleagues[53] found younger age, female sex, negative marital status, long working hours, and low reported job satisfaction to be predictive of burnout syndrome across the literature. Participation in wellness programs was related to lower burnout incidence. Although causation was not established because of limited number of longitudinal studies, the use of this information to increase preventive measures and guide interventions is recommended.

Every individual has a personal story and personal journey well before entering medical school and subsequent training. Personal histories including loss, trauma, physical and/or emotional abuse, and psychological distress before entering medical school and the stress of careers in medicine and surgery all contribute to the high occupational risk of suicide in physicians. Even strong support networks do not guarantee immunity against circumstantial and unanticipated crisis. Physicians are not superhuman. It is not only expected but anticipated that periodic help from a mental health professional will be needed to help optimize work-life integration and facilitate and protect their well-being.

PEER SUPPORT

Research has shown that men and women may need different kinds of networking to succeed.[1] The researchers reviewed types of networks that helped new male and female MBAs (Master of Business Administration) land executive leadership positions. They found that men benefit from being central in the networks and by being connected to multiple hubs of people with many contacts across different groups. Women required dual networks to land top positions. In addition to centrality, they also had to have an inner circle of close female contacts, despite having similar qualifications to men, including education and work experience.

Peer support may be experienced differently between men and women. Peer support can be most constructive and insightful if it occurs across genders and includes members representing the greatest diversity in all areas of professional and personal experience. Particularly relevant in health care is for hospitals to invest and create a formal peer support/second-victim program.

The Joint Commission boldly announced in 2020 a shift in focus to emphasize worker well-being, including blogs on establishing clinician well-being as a national priority, and removing mental barriers to mental health care for clinicians.[54] A formal peer support program in which investments are made to train various team members to become peer supporters, as well as senior leaders understanding how peer support positively affects quality and patient safety, is necessary to achieve the stated goals of focus on physician well-being and achieving zero harm. Dr Susan Scott (Scott and colleagues[55]) published in 2010 on "Caring for Our Own: Deploying a Systemwide Second Victim Rapid Response Team," She is a leading researcher who has published on the impact of peer support on patient safety for the Joint Commission.

The most critical factor in creating change to ensure fair, just, equitable, and inclusive environments is the intentional creation of a culture that affirms these values. Words matter. Conversations create change and define culture. Peer support across

not only small groups but entire tiers of faculty and leaders can collectively create a culture of shared advocacy, sponsorship, and bidirectional mentoring and relationships founded on trust and mutual respect.

SUMMARY

What has never been formally taught in medical school or subsequent training in a career in medicine is the fact that providing health care to others does not provide immunity against physical and/or mental illnesses or burnout. Intentional strategies at the individual, organizational, and systems levels must be used to encourage healthy work-life integration. Strategic recovery must occur on a daily basis. Normalizing use of mental health support, sharing vulnerabilities, leveraging peer support, and leveraging daily interactions to create a just and equitable health care culture are all critical components of true physician wellness.

DISCLOSURE

None.

REFERENCES

1. Available at: https://hbr.org/2019/02/research-men-and-women-need-different-kinds-of-networks-to-succeed.
2. Tawfik DS, Profit J, Morgenthaler TI, et al. Physician burnout, well-being, and work unit safety grades in relationship to reported medical errors. Mayo Clin Proc 2018;93(11):1571–80.
3. Wallace JE, Lemaire JB, Ghali WA. Physician wellness: a missing quality indicator. Lancet 2009;374(9702):1714–21.
4. Wei, JL. Individual and system approaches to physician/provider wellbeing. Bailey's.
5. Maslach C, Leiter MP. Understanding the burnout experience: recent research and its implications for psychiatry. World Psychiatry 2016;15(2):103–11.
6. Available at: https://globalwellnessinstitute.org/what-is-wellness/.
7. Available at: https://www.cdc.gov/hrqol/wellbeing.htm.
8. Available at: https://www.merriam-webster.com/dictionary/balance.
9. Available at: https://www.merriam-webster.com/dictionary/integration.
10. Available at: https://haas.berkeley.edu/human-resources/work-life-integration/.
11. Gade L, Yeo HL. "Work–Life Integration and Time Management Strategies. Clin Colon Rectal Surg 2019;32(6):442–9.
12. Available at: https://www.acgme.org/What-We-Do/Initiatives/Physician-Well-Being.
13. Raja S, Stein SL. Work-life Balance: History, Costs, and Budgeting for Balance. Clin Colon Rectal Surg 2014;27(2):71–4.
14. Restauri N, Sheridan AD. Burnout and Posttraumatic Stress Disorder in the Coronavirus Disease 2019 (COVID-19) Pandemic: Intersection, Impact, and Interventions. J Am Coll Radiol 2020;17(7):921–6.
15. Bajaj AK. Work/Life Balance: It Is Just Plain Hard. Ann Plast Surg 2018;80(5S Suppl 5):S245–6.
16. American Psychiatric Association. Diagnostic and statistical manual of mental disorders. 5th edition. Washington, DC; 2013.

17. Preti E, Di Mattei V, Perego G, et al. The Psychological Impact of Epidemic and Pandemic Outbreaks on Healthcare Workers: Rapid Review of the Evidence. Curr Psychiatry Repport 2020;22:43.
18. Prins JT, van der Heijden FMMA, Hoekstra-Weebers JEHM, et al. "Burnout, Engagement and Resident Physicians' Self-Reported Errors. Psychol Health Med 2009;14(6):654–66.
19. Bayham J, Fenichel EP. Impact of school closures for COVID-19 on the US healthcare workforce and net mortality: a modelling study. Lancet Public Health 2020; 5(5):e271–8.
20. Traylor AM, Tannenbaum SI, Thomas EJ, et al. Helping healthcare teams save lives during COVID-19: Insights and countermeasures from team science. Am Psychol 2020;76(1):1–13.
21. Bowe SN, Villwock JA. Does gender impact personality traits in female versus male otolaryngology residents and faculty? Am J Surg 2020;220(5):1213–8.
22. Dyrbye LN, Shanafelt TD, Balch CM. Daniel Satele, Jeff Sloan, and Julie Freischlag. "Relationship between Work-Home Conflicts and Burnout among American Surgeons: A Comparison by Sex. Arch Surg 2011;146(2):211–7.
23. Jolly S, Griffith KA, DeCastro R, et al. Gender Differences in Time Spent on Parenting and Domestic Responsibilities by High-Achieving Young Physician-Researchers. Ann Intern Med 2014;160(5):344–53.
24. Lyu HG, Davids JS, Scully RE, et al. Association of domestic responsibilities with career satisfaction for physician mothers in procedural vs nonprocedural fields. JAMA Surg 2019;154(8):689–95.
25. Thompson WT, Cupples ME, Sibbett CH, et al. Challenge of culture, conscience, and contract to general practitioners' care of their own health: qualitative study. Br Med J 2001;323(7315):728–31.
26. McKevitt C, Morgan M, Dundas R, et al. Sickness absence and 'working through' illness: a comparison of two professional groups. J Public Health Med 1997; 19(3):295–300.
27. Baldwin PJ, Dodd M, Wrate RM. Young Doctors' Health-II. Health and Health Behaviour. Soc Sci Med 1997 Jul;45(1):41–4.
28. Available at: https://hbr.org/2019/06/research-women-score-higher-than-men-in-most-leadership-skills.
29. Lautenberger D, Raezer C, Bunton SA. The Underrepresentation of Women in Leadership Positions in U.S. Medical Schools. Analysis in Brief. AAMC 2015;15(2).
30. Carr PL, Ash AS, Friedman RH. Faculty Perceptions of Gender Discrimination and Sexual Harassment in Academic Medicine. Ann Intern Med 2000;132(11): 889–96.
31. Sarsons H. Interpreting signals in the labor market: evidence from medical referrals [job market paper]. Boston (MD): Harvard University; 2017. Available at: https://scholar.harvard.edu/sarsons/publications/interpreting-signals-evidence-medical-referrals.
32. Torres MB, Salles A, Cochran A. Recognizing and Reacting to Microaggression in Medicine and Surgery. JAMA Surg 2019;154(9):868–72.
33. Pierce CM. Black psychiatry one year after Miami. J Natil Med Assoc 1970;62(6): 471–3.
34. Espaillat A, Panna DK, Goede DL, et al. An exploratory study on microagressions in medical school" What are they are why should we care? Perspec Med Edu 2019;8(3):143–51.

35. Solorzano D, Ceja M, Yosso T. Critical race theory, racial microaggression, and campus racial climate: The experiences of African American College Students. J Negro Educ 2001;69(1/2):60–73.
36. Periyakoil VS, Chaudron L, Hill EV, et al. Common types of gender-based microaggressions in medicine. Acad Med 2002;95(3):450–7.
37. Ganote C, Cheung F, Souza T. Don't remain silent!: strategies for supporting yourself and your colleagues via microresistances and ally development. Available at: http://www.pamelaroy.net/uploads/5/0/8/2/50825751/pod15dcwhitepaper.pdf.
38. Souza T. Responding to microaggressions in the classroom. Available at: https://www.facultyfocus.com/articles/effective-classroom-management/responding-to-microaggressions-in-the-classroom/.
39. Scully M, Rowe M. Bystander training within organizations. J Int Ombudsman Assoc 2009;2(1):1–9. Available at: https://studentsuccess.unc.edu/files/2015/10/Scully-and-Rowe-2009.pdf.
40. Fessell D, Cherniss C. Coronavirus Disease 2019 (COVID-19) and Beyond: Micropractices for Burnout Prevention and Emotional Wellness. J Am Coll Radiol 2020;17(6):746–8.
41. Lieberman MD, Eisenberger NI, Crockett MJ, et al. Putting Feelings Into Words. Psychol Sci 2007;18(5):421–8.
42. Available at: https://www.cnvc.org/training/resource/feelings-inventory.
43. Emmons RA, McCullough ME. Counting blessings versus burdens: an experimental investigation of gratitude and subjective well-being in daily life. J Pers Soc Psychol 2003;84(2):377–89.
44. Schimmack U, Reisenzein R. Cognitive processes involved in similarity judgments of emotions. J Pers Soc Psychol 1997;73(4):645–61.
45. Sexton JB, Adair KC. Forty-Five Good Things: A Prospective Pilot Study of the Three Good Things Well-Being Intervention in the USA for Healthcare Worker Emotional Exhaustion, Depression, Work-Life Balance and Happiness. Br Med J Open 2019;9(3):e022695.
46. McAllister-Williams RH. Do antidepressants work? A commentary on "Initial severity and antidepressant benefits: a meta-analysis of data submitted to the Food and Drug Administration" by Kirsch et al. Evid Based Ment Health 2008;11(3):66–8.
47. Krasner MS, Epstein RM, Beckman H, et al. Association of an Educational Program in Mindful Communication with Burnout, Empathy, and Attitudes among Primary Care Physicians. JAMA 2009;302(12):1284–93.
48. Available at: https://hbr.org/2020/09/when-your-boss-doesnt-respect-your-family-commitments.
49. Winston J, Johnson C, Wilson S. Barriers to Healthy Eating by National Health Service (NHS) Hospital Doctors in the Hospital Setting: Results of a Cross-Sectional Survey. BMC Res Notes 2008;1:69.
50. Available at: https://tinyfeet.co/on-the-blog/blood-sugar.
51. Available at: https://www.health.harvard.edu/blog/fertility-and-diet-is-there-a-connection-2018053113949.
52. Clough BA, March S, Chan RJ, et al. Psychosocial interventions for managing occupational stress and burnout among medical doctors: a systematic review. Syst Rev 2017;6:144.
53. Amoafo E, Hanbali N, Patel A, et al. What are the significant factors associated with burnout in doctors? Occup Med 2015;65(2):117–21.

54. Available at: https://www.jointcommission.org/resources/news-and-multimedia/blogs/dateline-tjc/2020/08/12/clinician-peer-support-programs-live-the-safe-and-sound-mission-in-2020/.
55. Scott SD, Hirschinger LE, Cox KR, et al. Caring for our own: deploying a system-wide second victim rapid response team. Joint Comm J Qual Patient Saf 2010;36(5):233–40.

Printed and bound by CPI Group (UK) Ltd, Croydon, CR0 4YY
03/10/2024
01040403-0013